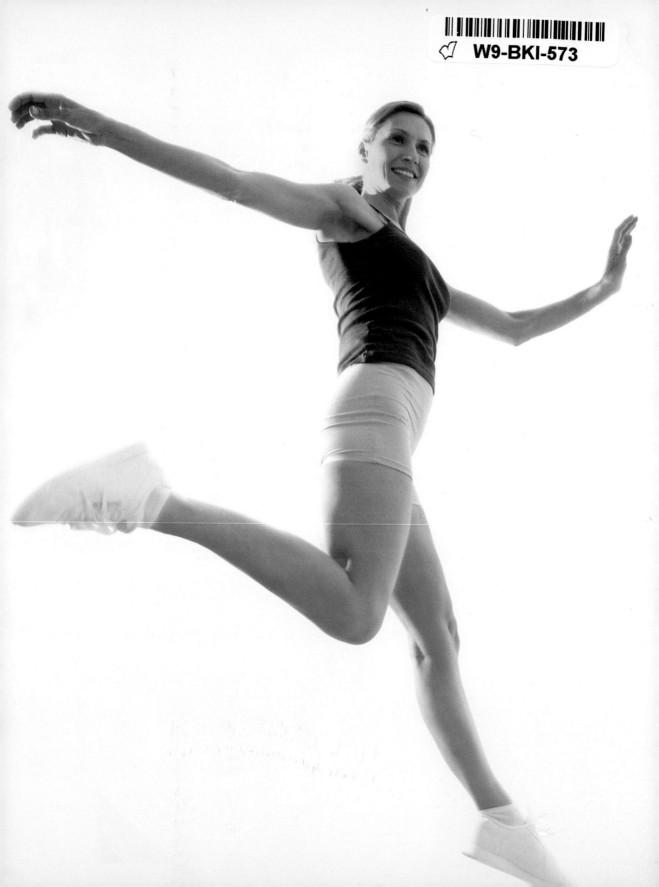

W9-BKI-573

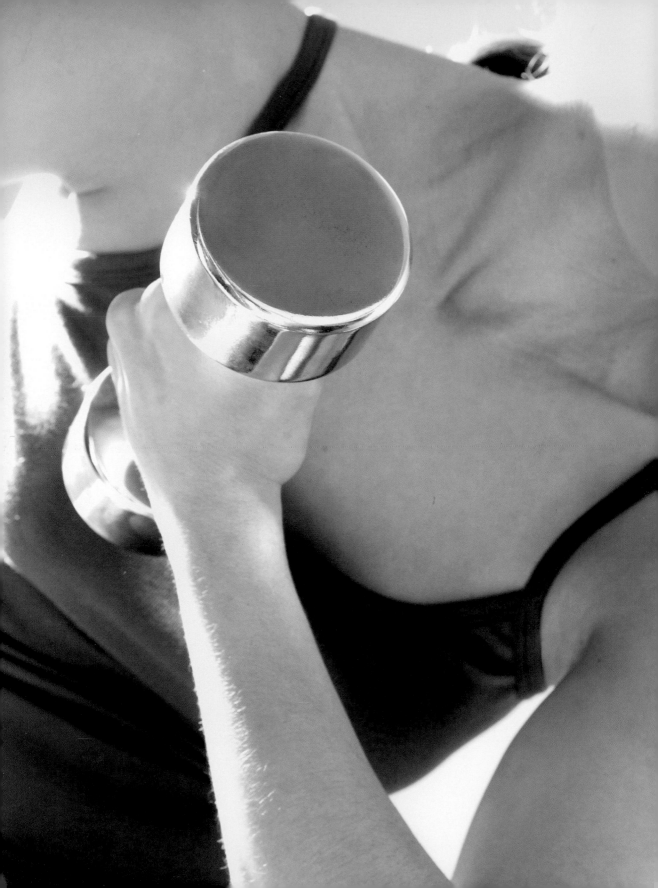

8 Weeks to a Younger Body

The at-home workout for a firmer, fitter you

JOAN PAGANO

London, New York, Melbourne, Munich, and Delhi

For James

Project Editor Irene Lyford
Project Art Editor Miranda Harvey
Senior Editor Jennifer Latham
Senior Art Editor Peggy Sadler
Managing Editor Penny Warren
Managing Art Editor Marianne Markham
Publishing Manager Gillian Roberts
Publishing Director Mary-Clare Jerram
Styling and Design Assistance Vicky Read
DTP Designer Sonia Charbonnier
Production Controller Rebecca Short

First American Edition 2007
07 08 09 10 11 9 8 7 6 5 4 3 2 1

Published in the United States by DK Publishing
375 Hudson Street
New York, New York 10014

Copyright © 2007 Dorling Kindersley Limited
Text copyright © 2007 Joan Pagano

All participants in fitness activities must assume the
responsibility for their own actions and safety. If you have
any health problems or medical conditions, consult with
your physician before undertaking any of the activities set
out in this book. The information contained in this book
cannot replace sound judgement and good decision
making, which can help reduce risk of injury.

All rights reserved under International and Pan-
American Copyright Conventions. No part of this
publication may be reproduced, stored in a retrieval
system, or transmitted in any form or by any means,
electronic, mechanical, photocopying, recording, or
otherwise without the prior written permission of the
copyright owners.

Cataloging-in-Publication data is available from
the Library of Congress
ISBN 978-0-7566-2600-6

Printed and bound by Tien Wah Press, Singapore
Color reproduction by Colourscan, Singapore

Discover more at
www.dk.com

CONTENTS

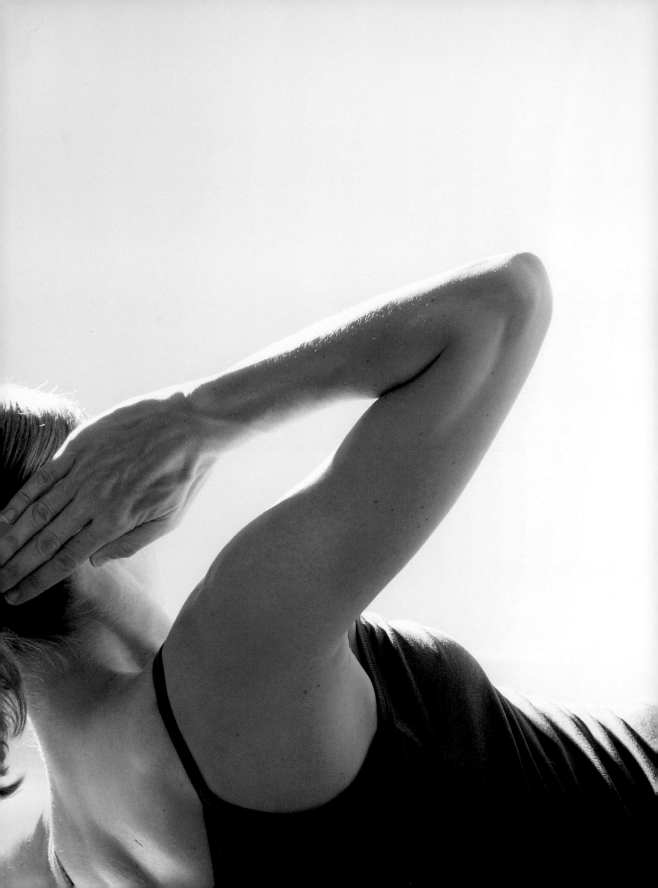

Take a moment to contemplate the process of renewal that you are about to begin with this program... Imagine feeling younger in body and spirit, empowered by achieving your goals.

before
you begin

CHANGING **BODIES...**

Inevitably, things change: you notice a little chunk at the waist that's affecting the way your clothing fits; you feel a bit stiffer in the mornings; you look for escalators instead of taking the stairs; a glimpsed reflection in a window reveals you're not as straight as you thought. We've all had moments of awareness when we realize we could be doing better.

Are you too old for your age?

Without regular exercise, your body ages faster than necessary. What makes us old are the physical limitations that restrict our capacity for life. Each of us wants to be able to maintain all of our everyday activities without undue fatigue and with energy to spare. Your ability to handle the physical demands of your daily life reflects your body's age (otherwise known as your functional age). Although genetics plays a role in retaining a youthful body, the single most important lifestyle factor is your engagement in a well-rounded exercise program.

Turning back the body clock

Two decades of working as a personal trainer has convinced me that we can turn back the body clock. I was in my thirties when I became interested in fitness, both personally and professionally. With years of high-school and college athletics a distant memory, and a career in the high-stress restaurant business in New York City taking its toll, at age 35 I felt more like 45 and my sense of well-being was suffering. A friend suggested yoga.

Little did I know that this was just the first step on the path that was unfolding before me, one that would lead to more personal growth and a change of career. I couldn't learn fast enough and soon earned my credentials and took the plunge. I loved it all—strength training, stretching, aerobics classes, a little running. The running began innocently enough, but culminated in my completing seven marathons in five years. Concern about the risk of overuse injuries and their

potential long-term effects, however, convinced me to return to a more moderate, balanced exercise program. Diligence, fine-tuning, and knowing personal limits are the other parts of the formula for success.

Age is no barrier

My clients are an inspiration to me and are living proof that fitness gives you an edge. Ranging in age from 14 to 94, they are at all levels of fitness and in various states of health. What they have in common is that each one of them strives to maintain her personal high-level performance and knows that her training program is fundamental to achieving this. Whether a top-level executive, a high-school student, an energetic mother, a breast-cancer survivor, or an active retiree, they are all dedicated to their fitness routines.

Revitalizing your body

With the help of this book, you will get the tools you need to revitalize your body. The first step is to discover your body's functional age. This is done by using a series of simple tests and measurements that you can carry out at home (see pp12–23). The results will help you assess your current level of fitness and identify your strengths and weaknesses in the three essential areas of exercise: cardiovascular fitness, muscle strength and endurance, and flexibility. By comparing your results with those of other women of your age, you will see how you measure up (see pp24–27).

This self-evaluation will guide you into a customized training program that is tailored to your current level of fitness. By following it for eight weeks, you can expect to improve your body age by developing muscle strength, losing body fat, gaining flexibility, and increasing your cardiovascular stamina.

The degree to which you can turn back your body clock depends in part on your starting level of fitness. If your starting level is below average for your age group, you stand to make the greatest initial improvements when you begin your exercise program.

Those whose starting level is above average can also improve their fitness profile and "get younger" by meeting the assessment standards for younger age groups. The more time you commit to your program, the more dramatic you can expect your results to be. As you become more fit and continue following programs for increasingly younger age groups, you can literally "drop a decade."

Fitness has changed my body and my life: a balanced exercise program can change yours, too. Your body age represents a quality of life—your chronological age is just a number.

To obtain maximum benefit and prevent *injury, careful attention to form and posture is essential when exercising.*

HOW TO USE THE BOOK

Designed to help you turn back your body clock with a personalized exercise program, this book follows a simple sequence of evaluating your current levels of fitness and exercise routines; comparing your fitness levels—as indicated by the results of your assessment tests—to norms for women in your age group; then directing you to the relevant resistance, flexibility, and cardio programs for your specific needs.

1 The first step is to assess your current levels of fitness with questionnaires that identify your exercise habits, your body-fat patterns, and any medical factors that could affect your ability to embark on an exercise program (*see pp12–17*).

The questionnaire on page 13 assesses your current activity levels in three areas of fitness: cardio, muscle strength, and flexibility

Your scores on this questionnaire will help pinpoint your strengths and weaknesses, and indicate where you need to concentrate your work

2 Then we invite you to take five tests that will enable you to check your fitness against norms for your age group. The tests cover cardio (*pp18–19*), muscle strength (*pp20–21*), and flexibility (*pp22–23*).

After each test, note your score in the box provided. Here, cardio fitness is assessed by taking the pulse before and after exercise (*see pp18–19*)

HOW DO YOU **RATE?**

It is very useful to have objective information on your initial level of fitness. Along with your health and medical information, your fitness profile defines your goals in an exercise program. Establishing a baseline also enables you to measure your improvement. Be sure to set realistic goals that you can meet as this will provide incentive to keep exercising.

How do you compare?

When you've completed the five assessment tests, go to the results chart for your age group (opposite and p26) and check your scores for each test against the norms. This will tell you how your current fitness levels compare with those of other women in your age group. Comparing your scores to the norms will also pinpoint your strengths and weaknesses in each of the three areas of fitness and allow you to tailor your exercise program precisely to your needs.

Keep a note of your starting fitness levels in the chart below, and after following your programs for eight weeks, take the tests again. You will then be able to see how far you have progressed toward your goal of achieving a younger body.

But don't stop there! Once you have seen the rejuvenating benefits of regular exercise, you are sure to want to continue, re-taking the tests after an eight-week period, and progressing to a younger-age program and more advanced level of exercise.

Using your test scores to determine your fitness program

For each of the fitness areas (Cardio, Resistance, Flexibility):

• **If you score Average,** begin with the program for your own age group.

• **If you score Above Average, Good, or Excellent,** you may start with the program for a younger age group.

• **If you score Below Average, Poor, or Very Poor,** begin with the program for an older age group.

Note: your fitness levels may not be the same in each area: for example, you may score Above Average in Cardio, Average in Resistance, and Below Average in Flexibility. In this case, you would follow the Cardio program for the age group younger than you; Resistance program for your own age; and Flexibility program for the age group older than you. If your score on the two tests for Cardio or Resistance indicate different fitness levels, choose the lower as your baseline.

	Cardio fitness		Resistance		Flexibility
	Resting heart rate	Step test	Crunches	Push-ups	Sit and reach
Your fitness level at start of program					
Your fitness level after 8 weeks					
Your fitness level after 16 weeks					

norms for women aged 26–35 (see Note on p27)

FITNESS LEVEL	Cardio Fitness		Resistance		Flexibility
	Resting heart rate page 18	Step test page 19	Crunches page 20	Push-ups page 21	Sit and reach pages 22–23
EXCELLENT	39–57	58–80	54–70	30–35	23–28
GOOD	60–62	85–92	44–50	26–29	21–22
ABOVE AVERAGE	64–66	95–101	37–41	21–25	20
AVERAGE	68–70	104–110	33–36	16–20	18–19
BELOW AVERAGE	72–74	113–119	28–32	10–15	16–17
POOR	77–81	122–129	22–26	5–9	14–15
VERY POOR	84–102	134–171	7–20	1–4	5–13

norms for women aged 36–45 (see Note on p27)

FITNESS LEVEL	Cardio Fitness		Resistance		Flexibility
	Resting heart rate page 18	Step test page 19	Crunches page 20	Push-ups page 21	Sit and reach pages 22–23
EXCELLENT	40–58	51–84	54–74	28–33	22–28
GOOD	61–63	89–96	42–48	23–27	20–21
ABOVE AVERAGE	65–67	100–104	35–38	18–22	18–19
AVERAGE	69–71	107–112	30–32	13–17	17
BELOW AVERAGE	72–75	115–120	23–28	8–12	15–16
POOR	77–81	124–132	19–22	4–7	13–14
VERY POOR	83–102	137–169	4–16	1–3	4–12

3 After completing the five tests, compare your scores with the norms for your age group. This will enable you to tailor your exercise program to your current fitness levels and to assess your progress after completing the programs.

After checking your test scores against the norms for your age group, enter your fitness level in each category on this chart and determine which programs you should follow

The results charts allow you to compare your score in each of the five tests against the norms for your age group, and to establish whether these are average, above average, or below average.

Each resistance exercise provides three levels of intensity to be worked through at your own pace

4 Guided by the results of your tests, follow the appropriate program in each of the three areas—resistance, flexibility, and cardio—for eight weeks. Then retake the assessment tests (see pp18–23) to see how far you have progressed.

In some of the exercises, an easier or more advanced alternative is shown as an inset feature

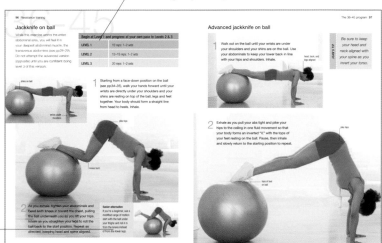

ARE YOU **FIT AND HEALTHY?**

You are totally in control of making positive lifestyle choices that determine your personal level of fitness and functional body age. Good fitness contributes to buoyant health, including feeling good, looking good, and enjoying life—in effect keeping you more youthful and upbeat as you age. But does being fit automatically mean that you are healthy; and, conversely, can you be healthy without being fit? In this section we examine such questions.

Cardiovascular stamina, muscular strength and endurance, flexibility, and body composition are the aspects of physical fitness that are most closely related to health. Each of these characteristics is directly related to good health and to your risk of developing certain types of disease—notably those that are associated with inactivity.

Benefits of cardiovascular fitness

A fit cardiovascular system is associated with a stronger heart muscle, slower heart rate, decreased chance of heart attack, and a greater chance of surviving if you do suffer a heart attack. Regular aerobic exercise can reduce your blood pressure and blood fats, including low density lipids (LDL), which can help you resist build-up of plaque in the arteries (atherosclerosis). It can also increase the protective high density lipids (HDL) and improve circulation and the capacity of the blood to carry oxygen throughout your body. Improving cardiovascular fitness also decreases your risk of some cancers (colon and possibly breast and prostate) and of obesity, diabetes, osteoporosis, depression, and anxiety.

Muscle strength and endurance

Muscular strength (the ability to exert force) and endurance (the ability of the muscles to exert themselves repeatedly) allow you to work more efficiently and to resist fatigue, muscle soreness, and back problems. Strengthening the muscles and joints allows you to increase the intensity and duration of

your cardiovascular training, enhancing your aerobic workouts and sports activities. As you work the muscles, you simultaneously stimulate the bones to build and maintain bone density, decreasing the risk of developing osteoporosis.

Stretching and flexibility

Your ability to stretch out the muscles and maintain range of motion in the joints is another aspect of muscular fitness. Stretching helps improve posture by correcting the tendency of certain muscles to shorten and tighten; it counteracts the physical stressors of our day-to-day activities and discharges tension from the muscles.

How does your routine rate?

A well-rounded exercise program has a definite structure and includes cardio, strength training, and stretching. The questionnaire opposite is based on the "FIT guidelines," which state that for exercise to be effective, it must be done with enough Frequency, Intensity, and for a long enough Time.

Frequency, or how often you perform the exercise, ranges from a minimum of two days (resistance training) to as many as six days (cardio) per week.

Intensity, or how hard you work, also depends on the component, but in general requires more exertion than normal to produce gains.

Time, or the length of your exercise session, varies according to the frequency and intensity, but in general must be at least 30 minutes to be effective.

SO YOU THINK YOU ARE FIT...

You may think you are fit because you go to the gym once or twice a week or play tennis on the weekends, but true fitness depends on a well-rounded exercise program that includes cardio work, strength training, and stretching. To rate your routine, look at the questions below and circle the answers that describe most accurately your actual physical activity over the past 6–8 months. Your answers will also highlight areas of fitness that you have been neglecting.

Cardio/aerobic exercise

Including brisk walking, jogging, running, jumping rope, biking, swimming, stair-climbing, step aerobics, aerobic dance, water aerobics, skating, cross-country skiing, dancing (e.g. line dancing, ballroom dancing), cardio boxing.

Frequency

- 5–6 times per week [1]
- 3 times per week [2]
- Less than once per week [3]

Intensity

- Sustained heavy breathing, perspiration [1]
- Moderate breathing and perspiration [2]
- Light breathing, no perspiration [3]

Time

- Over 30 minutes per session [1]
- 20–30 minutes per session [2]
- Less than 10 minutes per session [3]

Strength training

Including use of free weights, machines, stretch bands. A full-body workout should include performing 8–10 exercises that target the major muscle groups (legs, back, chest, shoulders, arms, abdomen), repeating each exercise 8–12 times.

Frequency

- 3 full-body workouts per week [1]
- 2 full-body workouts per week [2]
- 1 full-body workout per week or less [3]

Intensity

- Last few reps are somewhat difficult [1]
- Can complete 12–15 reps [2]
- Can easily complete more than 20 reps [3]

Time

- 2–3 sets per exercise, 8–12 reps per set [1]
- 1 set per exercise, 12–15 reps [2]
- 1 set per exercise, more than 20 reps [3]

Stretching

Including activities such as yoga and Pilates and other types of static stretching performed slowly and held for a period of time. Each stretch should target specific muscles used in your workouts for a total of 8–10 different body parts.

Frequency

- 4–7 days per week [1]
- 2–3 days per week [2]
- 1 day per week or less [3]

Intensity

- Sustained gentle pulling in target muscle [1]
- Gradual easing of stiff joints [2]
- Tightness and painful restriction [3]

Time

- 20–30 seconds per stretch [1]
- 10–15 seconds per stretch [2]
- 5 seconds per stretch [3]

To score:
Once you've answered every question, circling the numbers that correspond to your answers, add these numbers to find your overall score. Then check your score on the right to see how you rate. In addition, examine your answers in each category to see where your strengths and weaknesses lie, and use this information to guide your future exercise programs. Remember, the aim is all-round fitness.

0–9 Very active: you are optimizing your workout levels in all three categories and are prepared for an advanced level of training.

10–18 Satisfactory: you are meeting the basic recommendations for seeing results in all three categories and are at an intermediate level.

19–27 Inactive: if you are excelling in one category and ignoring the others, you need to work for balance. If you are not exercising at all, start gradually and build up in all areas.

Body composition and health

A lean, well-toned figure is something that most of us aspire to—and the ideal of a youthful body shape motivates many of us to go to the gym, sign up for fitness classes, and keep an eye on our diets.

But body composition and body shape are more than just about how we look: they are also closely related to fitness and health. With optimal body composition, including a high ratio of lean body mass to fat, you minimize your risk of developing diseases that are related to how body fat is distributed.

Are you an apple or a pear?

Studies show that a large waist circumference signals a greater risk of heart disease, high blood pressure, and diabetes than ample hips and thighs. (A waist measurement of 35in (89cm) or more is considered excessive for women, 41in (104cm) for men.) This relationship between body shape and disease is sometimes summed up by the concept of "apples and pears": a person who tends to gain weight around the middle is described as apple-shaped, while one whose

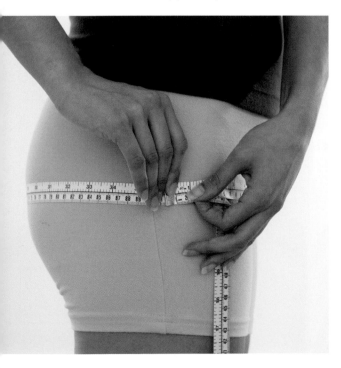

fat tends to settle around the hips and thighs is said to be pear-shaped. Unlike those who carry excess weight around the hips and thighs, people with apple-shaped figures are at increased risk of the diseases associated with abdominal obesity. Although your body type is inherited, you can minimize the associated health risks by controlling your weight and keeping fit.

Check your waist-to-hip ratio

Another simple way of determining body-fat distribution is the waist-to-hip ratio, which also relates to health risk. To determine your waist-to-hip ratio:
1 Measure your waist just above the belly button and below the notch in the center of the ribcage.
2 Measure around the maximal circumference of the buttocks.
3 Divide your waist measurement by your hip measurement to determine the ratio.
For example:
    Waist measurement = 30in (76cm)
    Hip measurement = 40in (102cm)
    Hip-to-waist ratio = 30 ÷ 40 (76 ÷ 102) = .75
Health risk increases with a high waist-to-hip ratio: in women aged 20–39, a ratio of more than .79 is considered high; for women aged 40–59, the figure is .82; and for those aged 60–69, it is .84.

Body mass index (BMI)

Based on a ratio of weight to height, BMI is used to assess the increased risk of weight-related health conditions. It may be inaccurate in some cases—for example, for someone with a lot of muscle mass, as muscle weighs more than fat—but the chart opposite is a simple and convenient way to check whether your weight is within healthy limits. If the result indicates that your weight poses health risk, seek advice from your medical practitioner.

Hip-to-waist ratio is a simple way to determine whether your body-fat distribution poses a health risk. Divide your waist measurement by your hip measurement to find the ratio.

CHECK YOUR BODY MASS INDEX (BMI)

Look down the column on the left-hand side of the table to find your weight (or the nearest to it); then look across that row until you see the column for your height. The number that appears where the two meet is your BMI score. To find out whether your score indicates that your weight is healthy for your height, go to the assessment underneath the table.

Weight	Height 58in (1.47m)	60in (1.52m)	62in (1.57m)	64in (1.62m)	66in (1.68m)	68in (1.73m)	70in (1.78m)	72in (1.83m)	74in (1.88m)	76in (1.93m)
120lb (54kg)	25	24	22	21	19	18	17	16	15	15
125lb (57kg)	26	24	23	22	20	19	18	17	16	15
130lb (59kg)	27	25	24	22	21	20	19	18	17	16
135lb (61kg)	28	26	25	23	22	21	19	18	17	16
140lb (63kg)	29	27	26	24	23	21	20	19	18	17
145lb (66kg)	30	28	27	25	23	22	21	20	19	18
150lb (68kg)	31	29	28	26	24	23	22	20	19	18
155lb (70kg)	32	30	28	27	25	24	22	21	20	19
160lb (73kg)	34	31	29	28	26	24	23	22	21	20
165lb (75kg)	35	32	30	28	27	25	24	22	21	20
170lb (77kg)	36	33	31	29	28	26	24	23	22	21
175lb (79kg)	37	34	32	30	28	27	25	24	23	21
180lb (82kg)	38	35	33	31	29	27	26	24	23	22
185lb (84kg)	39	36	34	32	30	28	27	25	24	23
190lb (86kg)	40	37	35	33	31	29	27	26	24	23
195lb (88kg)	41	38	36	34	32	30	28	27	25	24
200lb (91kg)	42	39	37	34	32	30	29	27	26	24
205lb (93kg)	43	40	38	35	33	31	29	28	26	25
210lb (95kg)	44	41	39	36	34	32	30	29	27	26
215lb (98kg)	45	42	39	37	35	33	31	29	28	26
220lb (100kg)	46	43	40	38	36	34	32	30	28	27
225lb (102kg)	47	44	41	39	36	34	32	31	29	27
230lb (104kg)	48	45	42	40	37	35	33	31	30	28
235lb (107kg)	49	46	43	40	38	36	34	32	30	29
240lb (109kg)	50	47	44	41	39	37	35	33	31	29
245lb (111kg)	51	48	45	42	40	37	35	33	32	30

What does your score mean?

Below 18.5	You are underweight, which may signal malnutrition
18.5–24.9	You are within a healthy weight range for your height
25–29.9	You are overweight, with an increased risk for health problems
30 and above	You are obese, with significantly increased risk for health problems

Can you be fit and unhealthy?

Even though the relationship between regular physical activity and good health is well established, it is important to understand that health and fitness are not always synonymous.

The assessment tests in this book (*see pp18–23*) evaluate your current level of fitness, not your state of health. Just because you score well on the 3-minute step test does not necessarily mean that you do not have heart disease: it is possible to have good aerobic endurance and still have heart disease. The only exercise test that can give you information about the health of your heart is a graded-exercise stress test, administered under the supervision of a cardiologist.

Conversely, just because you score poorly on the assessment tests does not mean that you are not healthy. Only your doctor can determine your state of health. If your clinical measures—such as your weight, blood pressure, cholesterol, and bone density—are within the normal range, then you are considered to be healthy. However, even small improvements in your fitness level can have significant health benefits.

Motivation and realistic goals

The assessments do, however, provide a valuable tool for establishing your baseline level of fitness and setting realistic goals. For those who have been lulled into blissful oblivion about not exercising, it can be a powerful motivator to actually see, in bald numbers, how you measure up against the norms for your age-group. I've had clients tell me it was like having a light shone in their eyes. For others, who are aware of how out-of-condition they are, it may be more appropriate to follow the 56–65 year old programs for eight weeks before taking the tests. For the athlete or dedicated exerciser, on the other hand, the assessments can provide fine-tuning for current training programs.

Before doing the tests

It is imperative that before undertaking any tests or exercises you complete the questionnaire opposite, which is designed to establish whether you should seek medical advice before starting an exercise program. The questions are principally designed to alert you to the symptoms of heart disease. There is one question that relates to orthopedic conditions (bone, joint or muscle injuries) that could be affected by exercise. If you have any of these, a physician can suggest appropriate exercise guidelines and restrictions or refer you to the proper health-care professional.

Diet and exercise are key to health and fitness: regular all-around exercise and a well-balanced, nutritious diet will keep you feeling good, looking good, and enjoying life to the fullest.

PHYSICAL ACTIVITY READINESS QUESTIONNAIRE—PAR-Q AND YOU

Regular physical activity is fun and healthy, and increasingly more people are starting to become more active every day. Being more active is very safe for most people. However, some people should check with their doctor before they start becoming much more physically active.

If you plan to become more physically active than you are now, start by answering the seven questions in the box below. If you are between the ages of 15 and 69, the PAR-Q will tell you if you should check with your doctor before you start. If you are over 69 years of age, and you are not used to being very active, check with your doctor.

Common sense is your best guide when you answer these questions. Please read the questions carefully and answer each one honestly: check YES or NO.

YES NO

☐ ☐ **1** Has your doctor ever said that you have a heart condition <u>and</u> that you should only do physical activity recommended by a doctor?

☐ ☐ **2** Do you feel pain in your chest when you do physical activity?

☐ ☐ **3** In the past month, have you had chest pain when you were not doing physical activity?

☐ ☐ **4** Do you lose your balance because of dizziness or do you ever lose consciousness?

YES NO

☐ ☐ **5** Do you have a bone or joint problem (for example, back, knee or hip) that could be made worse by a change in your physical activity?

☐ ☐ **6** Is your doctor currently prescribing drugs (for example, water pills) for your blood pressure or heart condition?

☐ ☐ **7** Do you know of <u>any other reason</u> why you should not do physical activity?

If you answered YES to one or more questions

Talk with your doctor by phone or in person BEFORE you start becoming much more physically active or BEFORE you have a fitness appraisal.
Tell your doctor about the PAR-Q and which questions you answered YES.
• You may be able to do any activity you want—as long as you start slowly and build up gradually. Or, you may need to restrict your activities to those which are safe for you. Talk with your doctor about the kinds of activities you wish to participate in and follow his/her advice.
• Find out which community programs are safe and helpful for you.

If you answered NO to all questions

If you answered NO honestly to all PAR-Q questions, you can be reasonably sure that you can:
• start becoming much more physically active—begin slowly and build up gradually. This is the safest and easiest way to go.
• take part in a fitness appraisal—this is an excellent way to determine your basic fitness so that you can plan the best way for you to live actively. It is also highly recommended that you have your blood pressure evaluated. If your reading is over 144/94, talk with your doctor before you start becoming much more physically active.

DELAY BECOMING MUCH MORE ACTIVE:
• if you are not feeling well because of a temporary illness such as a cold or a fever—wait until you feel better; or
• if you are or may be pregnant—talk to your doctor before you start becoming more active.

PLEASE NOTE:
If your health changes so that you then answer YES to any of the above questions, tell your fitness or health professional. Ask whether you should change your physical activity plan.

Informed Use of the PAR-Q: The Canadian Society for Exercise Physiology, Health Canada, and their agents assume no liability for persons who undertake physical activity, and if in doubt after completing the questionnaire, consult your doctor prior to physical activity.
Source: Physical Activity Readiness Questionnaire (PAR-Q) © 2002. Reprinted by permission from the Canadian Society for Exercise Physiology. http://www.csep.ca/forms.asp

TESTING **CARDIO FITNESS**

These two heart rate measures will give you an idea of your cardiovascular fitness. Resting heart rates normally range from 60–80 beats per minute, but in sedentary, poorly conditioned adults the rate may exceed 100bpm. Stressors such as exercise, anxiety, and caffeine also increase it. The step test measures your heart rate response to exercise. As your fitness level improves you can perform more work at relatively lower heart rates.

Resting heart rate

A strong heart can pump more blood with each beat, resulting in a lower heart rate both during exercise and at rest. A true resting heart rate is taken after a period of adequate rest. Count the first beat as "zero" and time yourself for 30 seconds. Multiply your score by two to arrive at the number of "beats per minute."

Your score
Enter your score here, then turn to pp24–27.

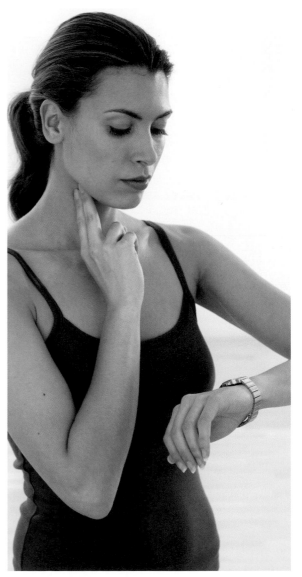

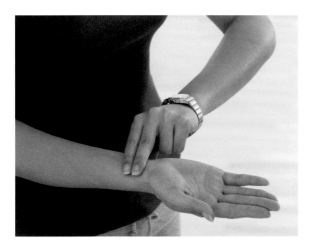

Taking your pulse at the wrist (the "radial pulse") Place your index and middle fingers on the palm-side of the opposite wrist, just above the thumb.

Taking your pulse at the neck (the "carotid pulse") Alternatively check the pulse in your neck, just below the jaw bone to the side of the larynx (voice box).

The step test

The three-minute step test measures your current level of aerobic conditioning by averaging your exercise and recovery heart rates. After exercise, your heart rate will begin to return to normal. The more fit you are, the faster your heart rate will recover from the stress of exercise. You will need a 12in- (30cm-) high step or bench and a watch with a second hand or digital display. If you begin to feel dizzy or nauseous while performing the test, stop immediately. Do not perform this test if you have serious balance issues.

Your score
Enter your score here, then turn to pp24–27.

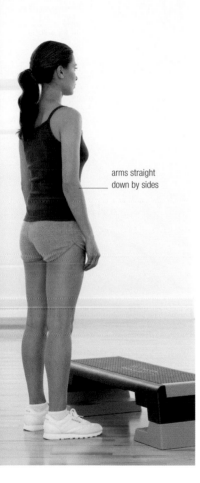

arms straight down by sides

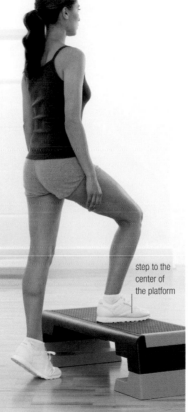

step to the center of the platform

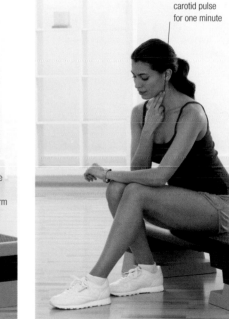

check your carotid pulse for one minute

1 Stand close to the step. To practice the correct pace, mark time in place at a rate of 24 step-cycles per minute (each cycle comprises right foot up, left foot up, right foot down, left foot down).

2 Begin stepping with the right foot, placing the entire foot on the platform. When stepping down, step onto the ball of the foot, then bring the heel to the floor. Avoid locking your knees while stepping.

3 Stop stepping after exactly three minutes. Sit on the step and locate your carotid pulse. Begin counting immediately and count for one full minute. Your score is your 60-second heart rate.

RESISTANCE **TESTS**

These tests assess your muscular endurance—or how many times your muscles can contract before fatiguing. Aging of the body is associated with disuse: muscles that are not used become weak, limiting your ability to lift, carry, push, and pull in your everyday activities. As you develop muscular strength and endurance, you turn back the body clock by increasing your stamina and work capacity.

The crunch test

This test, in which you curl your head and shoulders no higher than 30 degrees off the floor, measures the endurance of your abdominal muscles, important core stabilizers. The form for the test requires that the arms be extended to ensure a consistent range of motion. Before performing the test, measure 3½in (9cm) from the end of the mat and have a watch or timer ready to set for one minute.

Your score
Enter your score here, then turn to pp24–27

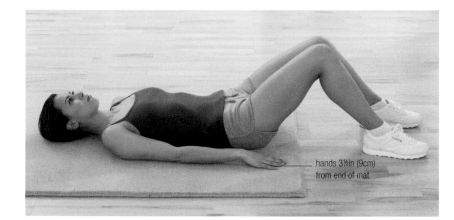

hands 3½in (9cm) from end of mat

1 Lie face-up on a mat, with your knees bent at 90 degrees and your feet flat on the floor. With your arms by your sides, palms down, position your hands 3½in (9cm) from the end of the mat.

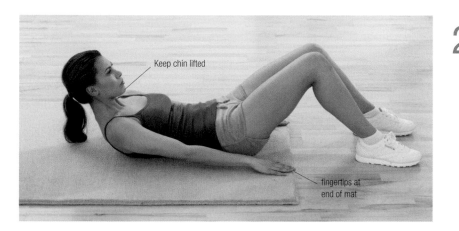

Keep chin lifted

fingertips at end of mat

2 Contract your abdominals and curl up, sliding your fingers forward to the end of the mat. Return to the starting position and repeat as many times as you can in one minute. Enter your score in the box above.

The push-up test

This test measures upper body endurance of the chest, shoulders, and triceps. In order to conform, you must use the modified position for this test push-up, with the knees as the pivotal point (even if you can do full-body push-ups). There is no time limit on this test, so do as many push-ups as you can while maintaining good form. Use your abdominals to keep your back straight while you lower your chest to the floor.

Your score
Enter your score here, then turn to pp24–27

1 Kneel on the mat with your hands shoulder-width apart, slightly ahead of your shoulders, and your lower legs resting on the mat. Shift your weight forward so there is no direct pressure on your knee caps.

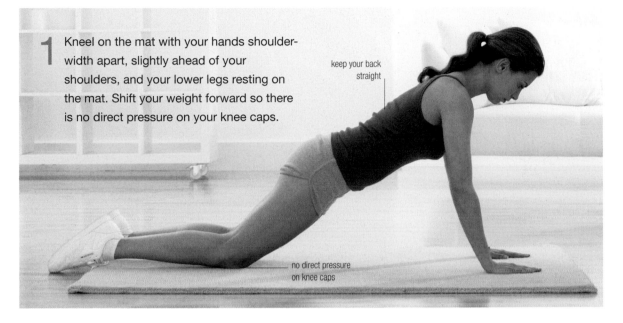

keep your back straight

no direct pressure on knee caps

2 Inhale as you bend your elbows, lowering your chest to the floor, until your chin touches the mat. Exhale as you push up to the starting position. Repeat as many times as you can, then enter your score in the box above.

FLEXIBILITY **TEST**

Technically, flexibility is a measure of the range of motion around a joint. It is determined by the "architecture" of the joint (the shape of the bones and cartilage) and the length of the muscles and ligaments crossing it. If range of motion is limited so the joint can't bend or straighten, it is said to be "tight" or "stiff." Being stiff is something we associate with old age, as it affects the way we look, the way we feel, and the way we move.

The sit-and-reach test

Although there is no single measure of total body flexibility, this test is commonly used in evaluation. It assesses hamstring and, to a lesser degree, lower back flexibility. As you perform the movement, take note of both the distance you reach on the tape-measure and how your spine moves. A flexible spine will curve forward fluidly from the low back to the upper back. If you are "stuck" in an upright posture as you reach forward, you should do a dedicated program of low back and hamstring stretching. Following the stretching program on pages 122–29 will help to increase your flexibility and improve your score. To reduce the risk of muscle strain, be sure to warm up first by doing a few minutes of walking or marching in place followed by a hamstring stretch, such as Step 1 below, or the one described on page 124.

Your score
Enter your score here, then turn to pp24–27

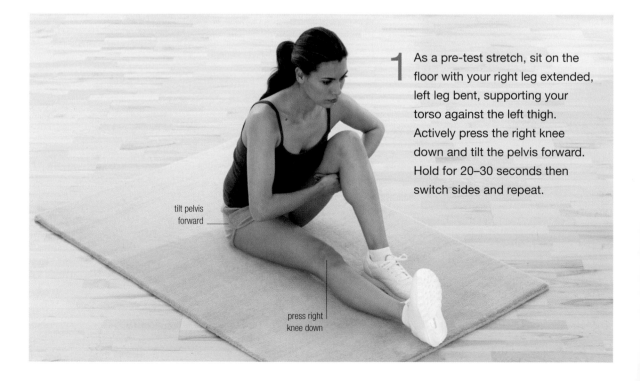

tilt pelvis forward

press right knee down

1 As a pre-test stretch, sit on the floor with your right leg extended, left leg bent, supporting your torso against the left thigh. Actively press the right knee down and tilt the pelvis forward. Hold for 20–30 seconds then switch sides and repeat.

2 Place a measuring tape with the 15in (38cm) mark at the edge of the mat, the "0" end toward you. Sit up straight with your heels at the edge of the mat, legs about 12in (30cm) apart. Extend your arms toward the tape, one hand on top of the other, so the middle fingers line up exactly.

heels at edge of mat

measuring tape with 15in (38cm) mark at edge of mat

3 Inhale, then as you exhale drop your head between your arms and slowly reach forward to touch the tape. Hold for 2 seconds, noting how far you have reached, then repeat. Enter your best score in the box opposite.

keep your knees straight

note how far your fingers reach

HOW DO YOU **RATE?**

It is very useful to have objective information on your initial level of fitness. Along with your health and medical information, your fitness profile defines your goals in an exercise program. Establishing a baseline also enables you to measure your improvement. Be sure to set realistic goals that you can meet as this will provide incentive to keep exercising.

How do you compare?

When you've completed the five assessment tests, go to the results chart for your age group (*opposite and p26*) and check your scores for each test against the norms. This will tell you how your current fitness levels compare with those of other women in your age group. Comparing your scores to the norms will also pinpoint your strengths and weaknesses in each of the three areas of fitness and allow you to tailor your exercise program precisely to your needs.

Keep a note of your starting fitness levels in the chart below, and after following your programs for eight weeks, take the tests again. You will then be able to see how far you have progressed toward your goal of achieving a younger body.

But don't stop there! Once you have seen the rejuvenating benefits of regular exercise, you are sure to want to continue, re-taking the tests after each eight-week period, and progressing to a younger-age program and more advanced level of exercise.

Using your test scores to determine your fitness program

For each of the fitness areas (Cardio, Resistance, Flexibility):

• **If you score Average**, begin with the program for your own age group.

• **If you score Above Average, Good,** or **Excellent**, you may start with the program for a younger age group.

• **If you score Below Average, Poor,** or **Very Poor**, begin with the program for an older age group.

Note: your fitness levels may not be the same in each area: for example, you may score Above Average in Cardio, Average in Resistance, and Below Average in Flexibility. In this case, you would follow the Cardio program for the age group younger than you; Resistance program for your own age; and Flexibility program for the age group older than you. If your score on the two tests for Cardio or Resistance indicate different fitness levels, choose the lower as your baseline.

	Cardio fitness		Resistance		Flexibility
	Resting heart rate	Step test	Crunches	Push-ups	Sit and reach
Your fitness level at start of program					
Your fitness level after 8 weeks					
Your fitness level after 16 weeks					

26-35 norms for women aged 26–35 (see Note on p27)

FITNESS LEVEL	Cardio Fitness		Resistance		Flexibility
	Resting heart rate page 18	Step test page 19	Crunches page 20	Push-ups page 21	Sit and reach pages 22–23
EXCELLENT	39–57	58–80	54–70	30–35	23–28
GOOD	60–62	85–92	44–50	26–29	21–22
ABOVE AVERAGE	64–66	95–101	37–41	21–25	20
AVERAGE	68–70	104–110	33–36	16–20	18–19
BELOW AVERAGE	72–74	113–119	28–32	10–15	16–17
POOR	77–81	122–129	22–26	5–9	14–15
VERY POOR	84–102	134–171	7–20	1–4	5–13

36-45 norms for women aged 36–45 (see Note on p27)

FITNESS LEVEL	Cardio Fitness		Resistance		Flexibility
	Resting heart rate page 18	Step test page 19	Crunches page 20	Push-ups page 21	Sit and reach pages 22–23
EXCELLENT	40–58	51–84	54–74	28–33	22–28
GOOD	61–63	89–96	42–48	23–27	20–21
ABOVE AVERAGE	65–67	100–104	35–38	18–22	18–19
AVERAGE	69–71	107–112	30–32	13–17	17
BELOW AVERAGE	72–75	115–120	23–28	8–12	15–16
POOR	77–81	124–132	19–22	4–7	13–14
VERY POOR	83–102	137–169	4–16	1–3	4–12

46-55 norms for women aged 46–55 (see Note opposite)

FITNESS LEVEL	Cardio Fitness		Resistance		Flexibility
	Resting heart rate page 18	Step test page 19	Crunches page 20	Push-ups page 21	Sit and reach pages 22–23
EXCELLENT	43–58	63–91	48–73	26–30	21–27
GOOD	61–64	95–101	37–44	21–25	19–20
ABOVE AVERAGE	65–69	104–110	33–36	16–20	17–18
AVERAGE	70–72	113–118	30–32	11–15	16
BELOW AVERAGE	73–76	120–124	25–28	6–10	14
POOR	77–82	126–132	19–23	3–5	12–13
VERY POOR	85–104	137–171	2–13	1–2	3–10

56-65 norms for women aged 56–65 (see Note opposite)

FITNESS LEVEL	Cardio Fitness		Resistance		Flexibility
	Resting heart rate page 18	Step test page 19	Crunches page 20	Push-ups page 21	Sit and reach pages 22–23
EXCELLENT	42–59	60–92	44–63	22–26	20–26
GOOD	61–64	97–103	35–42	17–21	18–19
ABOVE AVERAGE	65–68	106–111	27–32	12–16	16–17
AVERAGE	69–72	113–118	23–25	7–11	15
BELOW AVERAGE	73–77	119–127	18–22	5–6	13–14
POOR	79–81	129–135	11–15	3–4	10–12
VERY POOR	84–103	141–174	1–8	1–2	2–9

Maintaining fitness

If you are happy with your current fitness routine and the amount of time and effort it takes, you can "coast" for a while. The problem is that the body will adjust to a routine level of conditioning and you will need to change the program periodically to continue to get results. So even if your goal is maintenance, we recommend that after 12 weeks of doing the same exercises, you choose a different program in at least one area (cardio, strength, flexibility) to replace the one you have been doing. Continue to introduce a new component every 12 weeks.

Note: the norms for cardio fitness, crunch and flexibility tests were established by the YMCA, based on data from their members (*see p160*). Those for push-ups are an approximation, based on statistics compiled by a number of fitness organizations.

Comparing your test scores to the norms for your age group allows you to create a customized fitness program that is tailored precisely to your current levels of fitness.

Case study

Lucy, aged 53, has practiced yoga for years and is an advanced student. Now, however, she feels less limber, has gained a little weight around the middle, and is concerned to see her cholesterol level creeping up.

Predictably Lucy scored high in flexibility, but average on the resistance measures and below average in cardio. She will begin with the younger (36–45) stretching program, using the stability ball. She loves that it's similar to yoga, but will stretch muscles differently and includes a lot of moves to stretch the torso, which is where she feels stiff.

Since she scored average in resistance, she will stay in the 46–55 year program, which uses the step as its focus. This will stimulate her muscles as well as boost her cardio. For her main cardio program, she will start with the 56–65 walking program and work her way into the younger one. Cardio work will address Lucy's cholesterol levels, and, coupled with strength training, help to minimize weight gain.

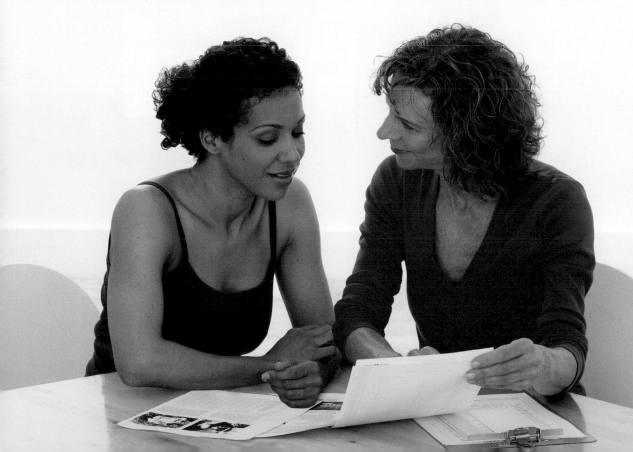

MUSCLES AND **EXERCISE**

If you know what muscle is working in a particular exercise, you can enhance your effort by mentally focusing on it. This will help you key into the muscular movement and improve your kinesthetic (body) awareness. The anatomical illustrations below and the glossary opposite will help you target specific areas that you want to work on—but remember that for a balanced workout, you need to work on all the major muscle groups.

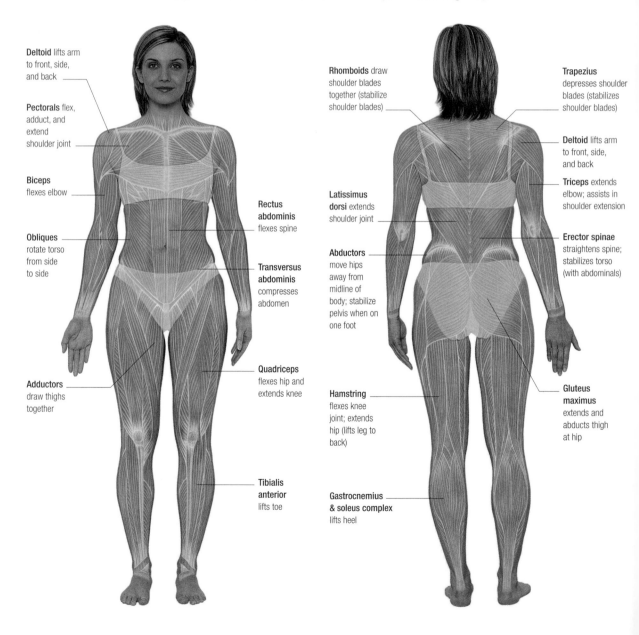

Deltoid lifts arm to front, side, and back

Pectorals flex, adduct, and extend shoulder joint

Biceps flexes elbow

Obliques rotate torso from side to side

Adductors draw thighs together

Rectus abdominis flexes spine

Transversus abdominis compresses abdomen

Quadriceps flexes hip and extends knee

Tibialis anterior lifts toe

Rhomboids draw shoulder blades together (stabilize shoulder blades)

Latissimus dorsi extends shoulder joint

Abductors move hips away from midline of body; stabilize pelvis when on one foot

Hamstring flexes knee joint; extends hip (lifts leg to back)

Gastrocnemius & soleus complex lifts heel

Trapezius depresses shoulder blades (stabilizes shoulder blades)

Deltoid lifts arm to front, side, and back

Triceps extends elbow; assists in shoulder extension

Erector spinae straightens spine; stabilizes torso (with abdominals)

Gluteus maximus extends and abducts thigh at hip

Muscles and targeted exercises

Abductors (outer thigh)
Back leg lift, p107
Balance clock, p65
Mini-squat with overhead press, pp104–5
Power-stepping, p45
Side squat with knee lift, p87
Side squat with weights, p66

Adductors (inner thigh)
Back leg lift on ball, p88
Plié with front shoulder raise, p108
Side squat with knee lift, p87
Side squat with weights, p66

Biceps (front of upper arm)
Biceps curl, p93
Concentration curl, p114
Double biceps curl, p54
Step-up with biceps curl, p61

Deltoid (shoulder: front, middle, rear)
Front and side shoulder raise, pp72–3
Knee-up with overhead reach, p67
Mini-squat with overhead press, pp104–5
Plié with front raise, p108
Reverse fly/shoulder extension, pp110–11
Shoulder flexion/extension, p53

Erector spinae group
Back leg lift, p107
Back leg lift on ball, p88
Bent-over alternating lat row, p109
Cross-body reach, intermediate, p49
Dead lift, p106
Front lunge with ball, p86
Jackknives on ball pp96–7
Kneeling triceps kickback, p113
Plank with knee bend, p79
Push/pull on ball, p95
Reverse fly/shoulder extension, pp110–11

Gastrocnemius & soleus complex (calf)
Calf raise, p70
Calf raise/heel drop, p50
Toe walking, p146

Gluteus maximus (buttocks)
Back leg lift, p107
Back leg lift on ball, p88
Balance clock, p65
Ball squat, p85
Cross-body reach, intermediate, p49
Dead lift, p106
Explosive chair stand, p44

Front lunge with ball, p86
Knee-up with overhead reach, p67
Lunge and narrow squat, pp68–9
Lunges, pp98–103
Lunge/squat combo, pp46–7
Mini-squat with overhead press, pp104–5
Plié with front shoulder raise, p108
Side squat with knee lift, p87
Side squat with weights, p66
Step-up sequence, pp58–64

Hamstring (back of thigh)
Back leg lift, p107
Back leg lift on ball, p88
Balance clock, p65
Ball squat, p85
Dead lift, p106
Explosive chair stand, p44
Front lunge with ball, p86
Lunge and narrow squat, pp68–9
Lunges, pp98–103
Lunge/squat combo, pp46–7
Mini-squat with overhead press, pp104–5
Side squat with knee lift, p87

Latissimus dorsi
Bent-over alternating lat row, p109
Lat pull-down, p51
One arm row, p71
Pullover on ball, p90
Reverse fly/shoulder extension, pp110–11
Seated lat row, p89
Shoulder flexion/extension, p53

Obliques (sides of waist)
Bicycle crunch, p77
Crunch and twist, p94
Dead bug, p78
Jackknives on ball, pp96–7
Plank with knee bend, p79
Push/pull on ball, p95
Torso twist with weight, pp116–17

Pectorals (chest)
Alternating chest press, p91
Chest fly, p75
Incline chest press, p52
Modified push-up, p74
Pullover on ball, p90
Push-up with a touch, p112
Reverse fly/shoulder extension, pp110–11
Shoulder flexion/extension, p53

Quadriceps (front of thigh)
Balance clock, p65
Ball squat, p85
Cross-body reach, intermediate, p49
Explosive chair stand, p44
Front lunge with ball, p86
Knee-up with overhead reach, p67
Lunge and narrow squat, pp68–9
Lunges, pp98–103
Lunge/squat combo, p46–7
Mini-squat with overhead press, p104–5
Plié with front shoulder raise, p108
Side squat with knee lift, p87
Side squat with weights, p66
Step-up sequence, pp58–64

Rectus abdominis (length of abdomen)
Basic crunch, p57
Bicycle crunch, p77
Crunch and twist, p94
Full crunch, p115
Jackknives on ball, pp96–7
Let-down, p56
Torso twist with weight, advanced, p117

Rhomboids & trapezius (between shoulder blades)
Bent-over alternating lat row, p109
Knee-up with overhead reach, p 67
Lat pull-down, p51
One arm row, p71
Seated lat row, p89
Triceps dip, p76
Triceps push-down, p55

Tibialis anterior (front shin)
Calf raise/heel drop, p50
Heel walking, p146

Transversus abdominis (deep abdominals)
Dead bug, p78
Jackknives on ball, pp96–7
Pelvic tilt, p122
Plank with knee bend, p79
Push/pull on ball, p95

Triceps (back of upper arm)
Triceps dip, p76
Triceps extension, p92
Triceps kickback, p113
Triceps push-down, p55

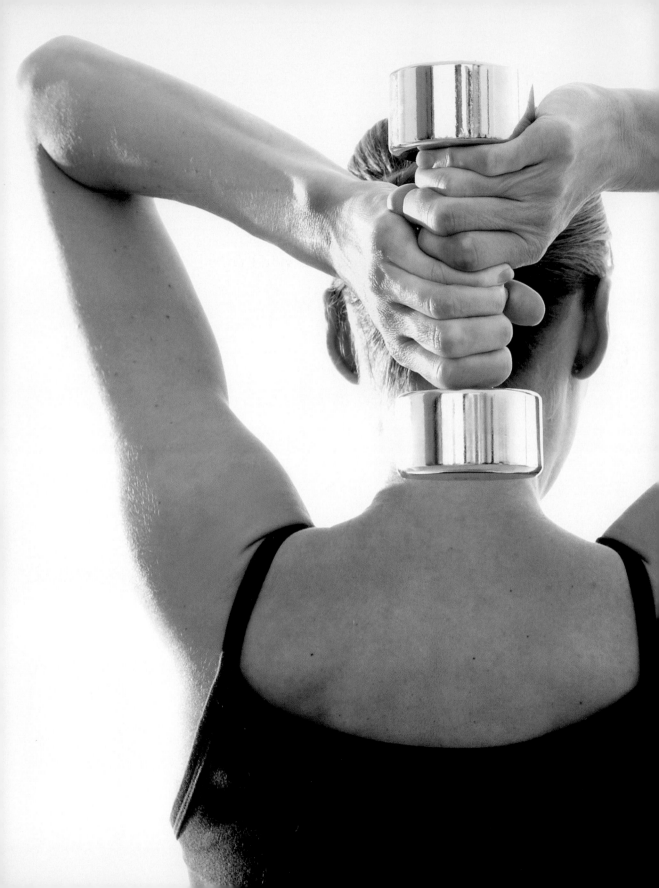

Strength training sculpts the contours of your body and strengthens the bones within. By building lean body mass, it boosts your metabolism and your energy levels, making you resistant to the slow down that occurs with age.

resistance
training

USING THE **EQUIPMENT**

All the equipment I have chosen for this book—stretch bands, step, stability ball, and free weights—is useful for in-home training. Each piece has its own benefits, and together they create a home-gym that is easy to store and offers a lot of variety in exercise choices. A mat is also useful to provide cushioning as well as traction for some of the exercises.

What to wear for your workout

Choose clothing that you can move in and wear supportive shoes that allow for movement in all directions. Cross trainers are a good choice for resistance training. Running and walking shoes are designed primarily to move forward and backward and are not a good choice for other exercises. (See page 146 for more advice about walking/running shoes.)

Get to grips with stretch bands

As a type of resistance equipment, bands are uniquely portable. They can be used for a full-body workout (*see The 56-65 program, pp44–57*) or as a complement to free-weight exercises when you want to target the same muscle in a different way. For example, if you want to focus on your triceps, do the appropriate exercise from your age-group program then add an extra triceps exercise using the band.

The level of resistance is determined by the band's thickness and is designated by different colors, which vary according to manufacturer. Buy a pack of three (light, medium, and heavy) or get at least two (light and medium if you are just beginning; medium and heavy if you are more experienced).

The bands can be a little tricky to use, but are well worth learning. Since more resistance occurs at the ends of the range of motion, try each exercise first without the band to establish your pain-free range. Anchor the band carefully before beginning each exercise and, as you work with it, keep width in the band to prevent it from sliding up the limb or digging into your skin.

Using stretch bands

Stretch bands usually come in 3-ft (90cm-) and 4-ft (1.2m) lengths. The longer one is more versatile, but the shorter length may be easier to use if you are tying it in a loop.

Holding the band

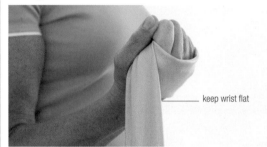

keep wrist flat

To grip the band, wrap it around the entire hand. When you are pulling on it, keep the band wide and be sure to keep your wrists in neutral alignment.

Tying the band around your legs

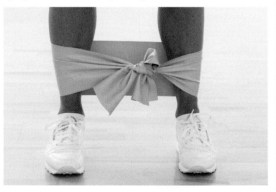

Tie the band with a half-bow, leaving one long end. Check that the bow is secure before beginning to exercise. If the skin on your legs is sensitive, wear socks or leggings to prevent irritation while you exercise.

To maintain the bands and preserve their elasticity, store them flat in a plastic baggie and powder them from time to time with baby powder or cornstarch. Make sure that you untie them if you have knotted them up for an exercise. Over time the bands will deteriorate, become tacky to touch, and may develop tiny holes and tears that can cause them to break during use. Examine them regularly for signs of wear. **Caution**: if you have carpal tunnel syndrome (a wrist injury associated with repetitive movements), do only those stretch-band exercises prescribed by a physician or physical therapist. If you have high blood pressure, use lighter resistance in a supervised program.

Stepping up the pace

The step itself is not a piece of resistance equipment, but it offers many benefits to your program as a tool for increasing cardio stamina, developing coordination, and conserving bone mass. You can perform consecutive minutes of stepping for an aerobic workout, and because it is specific to the Step test (see p19), doing this is the best way to improve your score on that test. Or you can combine weight-training exercises with 2–3 minutes of step intervals for an effective circuit training workout, the goal of which is to keep your heart rate elevated for at least 30 minutes.

Exercises that challenge your normal stepping patterns (*Alternating lead feet, p60*) or that combine upper and lower body movements (*Step-up with biceps curl, p61*) will help develop coordination by forging new neuromuscular pathways as your mind and body work together to master the moves.

As a potentially high intensity, low-impact exercise, stepping provides a safe, effective workout, maximizing intensity to the bones while minimizing stress to the joints. The intensity of the exercise depends on the height of the platform, the speed at which the steps are performed, and the amount of weight used.

Different models of steps are adjustable to different heights and have platforms of different sizes—some compact for storage, some larger for additional use as

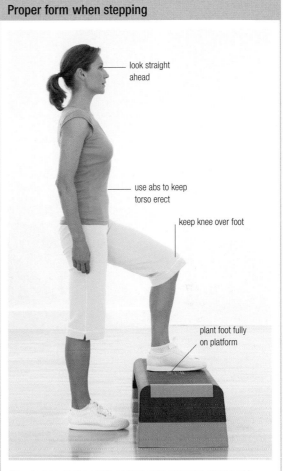

Proper form when stepping

look straight ahead

use abs to keep torso erect

keep knee over foot

plant foot fully on platform

Stand close to the platform and step onto the center of it with the entire sole of the foot. Step down on the ball of the foot and bring the heel to the floor. Avoid bending your knees less than 90 degrees while weight-bearing and be careful not to lock your knees at any time.

a bench for weight training. Choose a step with a range of 6–12in (15–30cm). The Step test requires a 12in- (30cm-) step, even though you may not use that height for your workouts. If you are beginning, start low at 6–8in (15–20cm). Be careful when assembling the step and check its stability before starting to step. **Caution**: if you have knee or lower back issues, test yourself by starting at a low height, slow speed, and without holding weights. If you have serious balance issues choose another type of program.

Using a stability ball

The stability ball (also called a Swiss ball) adds many advantages to your home fitness program, aiding in posture and core stability, motor control, balance and coordination, and stretching. Balls come in different sizes, represented by different colors, which vary by manufacturer. Your ball should be fitted to your particular body proportions. When sitting on the ball, your hips and knees should be bent at 90 degrees with your feet flat on the floor. If you have long legs or are of heavy proportions, you may need a larger ball. The following guidelines indicate the appropriate size of ball to choose, according to your height:

- 55–60in (1.4–1.5m)   18in (45cm) ball
- 61–66in (1.5–1.7m)   22in (55cm) ball
- 67–73in (1.7–1.8m)   26in (65cm) ball
- 74–80in (1.8–2m)   30in (75cm) ball
- over 81in (2m)   34in (85cm) ball

Getting onto the ball

Before using the stability ball in exercises, master the neutral sitting position (*bottom left*), then practice getting into prone and bridge positions; use the same progressions to get on and off the ball. Perform these movements slowly. They all require balance, core stabilization, and endurance, which may cause more fatigue than you realize at the time.

Establishing prone position

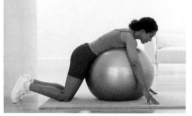

1 *Kneel on a mat, resting your abdomen on the ball, fingertips lightly touching the floor and toes tucked under.*

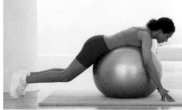

2 *Extend your legs, pushing your toes into the floor and rolling the ball under you as you start to move forward.*

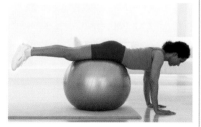

3 *Walk your hands forward, moving your torso away from the ball until your hips (or knees) are on the ball, feet in the air.*

Neutral sitting and adopting bridge position

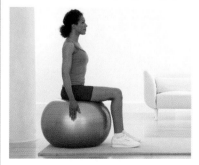

1 *Begin in neutral sitting position with your knees bent at 90 degrees and aligned over your ankles, arms straight down, your hands touching the sides of the ball.*

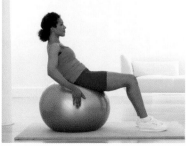

2 *Walk your feet forward and begin sliding down on the ball. If you are just learning, hold onto the sides of the ball to help you balance as you slide down.*

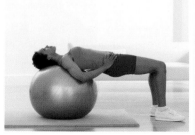

3 *Continue sliding down until your head, neck, and shoulders are supported. Use your glutes (see pp28–29) to lift your hips. Keep your knees over your ankles.*

To inflate your ball, use a manual pump that pumps high volumes of air at low pressure (bicycle pumps will generally not work). Never over-inflate the ball. If you are deciding between two sizes, choose the larger ball and slightly under-inflate it. A fully inflated ball is more resilient and more challenging to use.

When you inflate the ball for the first time, just inflate it to 80 percent capacity, wait 24 hours, then continue inflating to the proper size. This will extend the longevity of the ball.

Over time and with use the balls may lose a little air and need to be pumped up. Inspect the exterior of the ball regularly for any scrapes, scuffs, punctures, or tears that might cause air leakage.

Caution: If you have poor balance, use a stability ball only with the supervision of a trained professional.

Using free weights

Free weights, or dumb bells, are the most basic resistance equipment for the home. They make resistance training interesting by challenging your balance, coordination, and core stabilization. Since you lift them with individual limbs, it is easy to spot imbalances in the body and use them to improve symmetry. You can effectively isolate one muscle at a time, or combine movements to challenge whole muscle groups.

Made of solid metal, free weights may be covered in gray enamel, chrome, vinyl or neoprene (which contains latex), or rubber. Enamel and chrome coatings chip and flake over time, presenting a risk in use. Vinyl and neoprene coatings eliminate this risk, come in bright colors, and are nicer to hold.

Free weights are widely available in weight increments of 1-, 2-, 3-, 4-, 5-lb; or 0.5-, 1-, 2-, 3-, 4-, 5-kg, and so on. (**Note:** the conversions offered in this book are approximations.) You will need at least two pairs of free weights for your resistance work:

- Beginner: 3lb and 5lb (1kg and 2kg)
- Intermediate: 5lb and 8lb (2kg and 4kg)
- Advanced: 10lb and 12lb (5kg and 5.5kg).

Correct form when using weights

Concentrate on proper form and alignment, stabilizing the core body before you lift. Coordinate the movement with your breath: inhale first then exhale slowly as you lift the weight, controlling the pace with your breathing.

Holding the weight

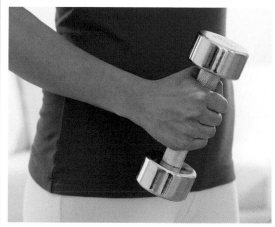

Be sure to keep the wrist flat (in neutral) to prevent any strain or injury to the joint. Avoid bending or "cocking" the wrist. Do not grip the weight too tightly.

Picking up the weights

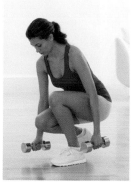 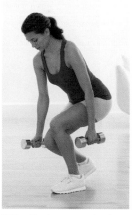

1 *Kneel down to the floor by bending your knees. Keep your back straight and tighten your abdominals as you prepare to lift the weights off the floor.*

2 *Use the large muscles in your legs to do the lifting, squeezing your glutes as you stand up. Keep working your abdominals to protect the lower back.*

UNIVERSAL **COOL-DOWN**

It is important to lengthen the muscles after having contracted them against resistance. This series of stretches provides an alternative to a more extensive flexibility program following your resistance training segment. It also provides good tension release at any time. Perform each of the stretches once and hold for three deep breathing cycles.

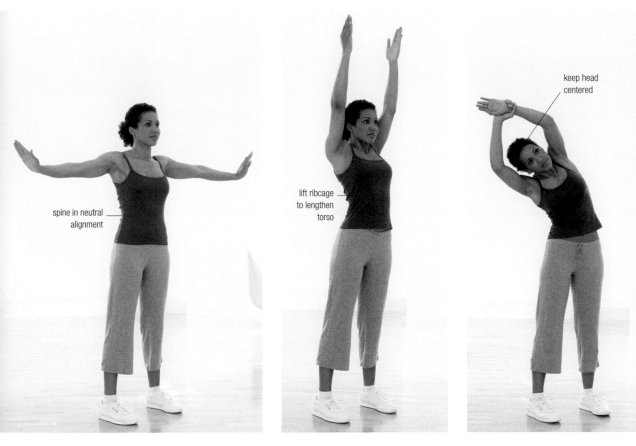

spine in neutral alignment

lift ribcage to lengthen torso

keep head centered

1 Chest and shoulder stretch: stand with your feet parallel, hip-width apart, knees soft. Extend your arms out to the sides just below shoulder level, palms facing out. Press your hands outward, as if you were pushing against two walls.

2 Lat stretch: stand as before, ribs stacked over hips. Draw the shoulder blades down and reach both arms up, palms facing in. Lengthen through the torso by lifting your ribcage.

3 Side stretch: take your left wrist in your right hand and pull your torso to the side, feeling the stretch all the way down to the left hip. Avoid twisting the torso. Repeat to the other side.

4 Spinal roll-down: from the standing position, with your arms by your sides, tuck your chin into your chest and begin rolling down one vertebra at a time. Allow your arms to come forward as you round your spine. Keep your knees soft.

5 Downward dog: from the above position, place your palms flat on the floor; walk your hands forward as you press your heels into the floor. Keep lengthening through the spine and reach up with your hips. (If necessary, bend knees slightly to release heels to floor.)

lengthen spine as you walk forward

press heels to floor

THE 56-65 **WARM-UP**

The warm-up prepares the body for the more strenuous work of the resistance training program. The rhythmic stepping patterns elevate the temperature of the core body and muscle tissue and bathe the joints in lubricating (synovial) fluid, while the arm movements rehearse the muscles most involved in the upper body strengthening exercises.

Marching in place

Toe tap to front

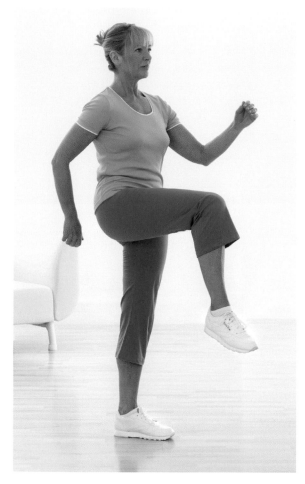

pump arms
energetically

tap toe
to front

Begin marching, lifting your knee up as high as you can and raising the opposite arm. Step down onto the ball of the foot, rolling through to the heel. Continue marching, using opposite arm/leg action.

• **Reps** Do 20 reps (one rep = both sides)

Continuing to march to the same rhythm, change the foot pattern by tapping the toes to the floor at the front, alternating feet. Continue pumping the arms in opposition as you march.

• **Reps** Do 20 reps (one rep = both sides)

Heel tap to front

Wide marching in place

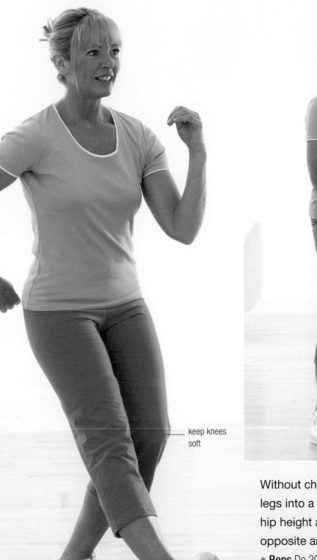

keep knees soft

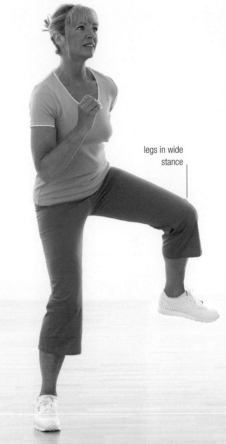

legs in wide stance

Without changing the rhythm, separate your legs into a wider stance and lift your knee to hip height as you march. Continue pumping opposite arms as before.

• **Reps** Do 20 reps (one rep = both sides)

Change the foot pattern to a heel tap to the front. Continue marching, alternating feet and arms. Pointing the foot (as in the last step) and flexing (as here) help to warm up the muscles of the lower leg.

• **Reps** Do 20 reps (one rep = both sides)

JOAN'S TIP

Pumping your arms energetically increases the benefit of the warm-up to your upper body.

Step-touch

1 Maintaining the same rhythm and continuing to pump the arms in opposition, change the foot pattern to a step-touch. Keep your knees soft as you shift your weight onto your left leg.

pump opposite arm

tap toe to floor

2 Bringing your right leg in to meet the left, tap the right toe to the floor; immediately step to the right and tap the left foot to the floor. Continue this pattern.
• **Reps** Do 20 reps (one rep = both sides)

Step-touch with lateral raise

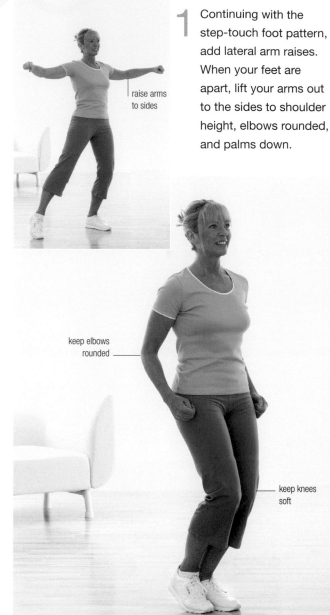

1 Continuing with the step-touch foot pattern, add lateral arm raises. When your feet are apart, lift your arms out to the sides to shoulder height, elbows rounded, and palms down.

raise arms to sides

keep elbows rounded

keep knees soft

2 When your feet are together, with the toes tapping the floor beside the opposite foot, lower your arms to your sides, with the elbows still rounded. Continue this pattern, synchronizing arm and leg movements.
• **Reps** Do 20 reps (one rep = both sides)

Step-touch with chest press

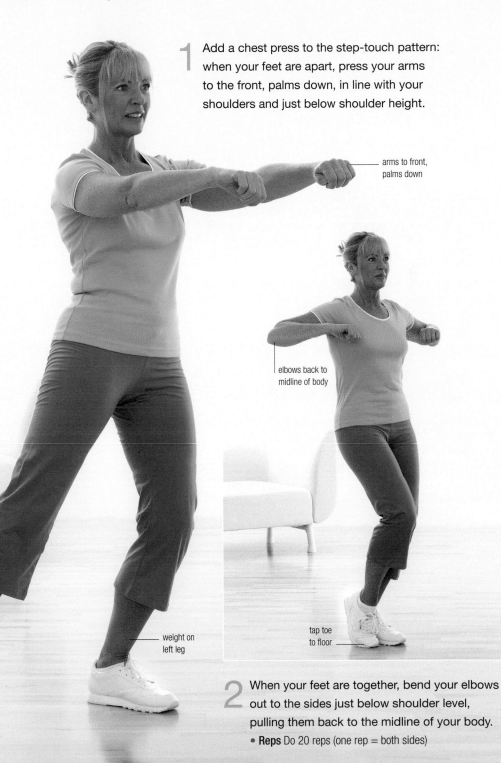

1 Add a chest press to the step-touch pattern: when your feet are apart, press your arms to the front, palms down, in line with your shoulders and just below shoulder height.

arms to front, palms down

elbows back to midline of body

weight on left leg

tap toe to floor

2 When your feet are together, bend your elbows out to the sides just below shoulder level, pulling them back to the midline of your body.

• **Reps** Do 20 reps (one rep = both sides)

Tap-back with lat pull

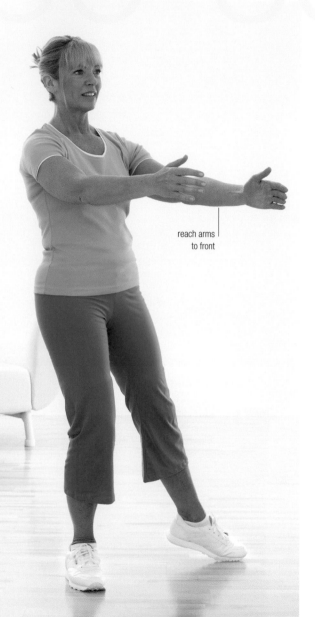

reach arms
to front

pull elbows
back, hands
to waist

tap toes
behind you

1 Without any interruption in your stepping, and maintaining the same rhythm, reach both arms forward above waist level, palms in, as you shift your weight to the right leg. Remember to keep your knees soft as you continue stepping.

2 Change the foot pattern, now crossing the left foot behind you and tapping the toes to the floor. At the same time, bend your elbows back, pulling your hands in to your waist. Repeat, tapping the right foot behind.
• **Reps** Do 20 reps (one rep = both sides)

Tap-back with biceps curl

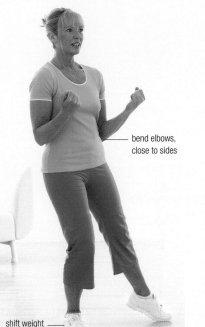

bend elbows, close to sides

arms down, palms forward

shift weight to right foot

1 Continue the foot pattern, tapping to the back, but change the arm movement to a biceps curl: when you shift your weight, switching sides, bend your elbows, keeping them close to your sides.

tap toes behind you

2 As you cross your foot behind you to tap to the floor, bring your arms down by your sides, palms facing forward. Continue this pattern, synchronizing arm and leg movements and maintaining the rhythm.
• **Reps** Do 20 reps (one rep = both sides)

Toe taps

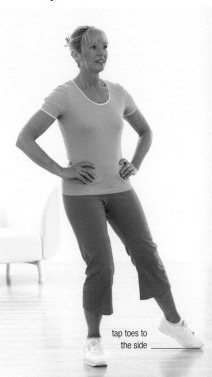

tap toes to the side

Complete the warm-up with toe taps. With your legs wider than hip-width apart, hands on your waist, shift your weight to your right leg and straighten the left leg out to the side, tapping the toe to the floor. Switch sides and repeat.
• **Reps** Do 20 reps (one rep = both sides)

JOAN'S TIP

At the end of your warm-up you should feel warm and start to break a light sweat.

THE **56–65** PROGRAM

Resistance training not only strengthens the muscles but also benefits the bones, helping to build bone density in the formative years and conserving bone mass in later years. Since the pull of the muscle on the bone has a localized loading effect, you must do exercises for all the major muscle groups in order to reinforce the entire skeleton.

Explosive chair stand

Performing this exercise with a burst of speed helps restore the fast twitch muscle fibers, which shrink with age, causing us to slow down. The exercise targets the large muscles of the upper leg for strength and stability and the thigh bone for improved bone density.

Begin at Level 1 and progress at your own pace to Levels 2 & 3	
LEVEL 1	10 reps, without band: 1–2 sets
LEVEL 2	12–15 reps, light or medium band: 1–2 sets
LEVEL 3	8–12 reps, heavy band; 2–3 sets

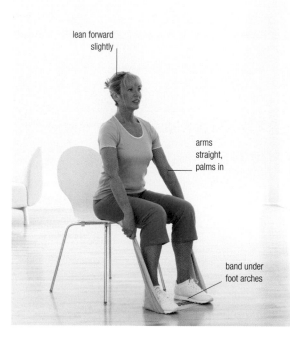

lean forward slightly

arms straight, palms in

band under foot arches

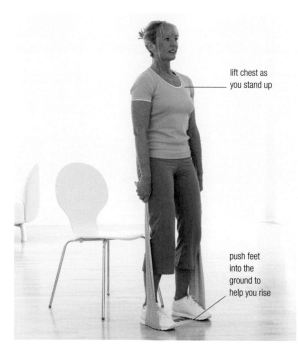

lift chest as you stand up

push feet into the ground to help you rise

1 Sit on the edge of a sturdy chair, holding the band as shown. Legs are hip-width apart, feet parallel, knees bent at right angles, directly over feet. Maintain tension in the band throughout.

2 Inhale, then exhale as you lean forward slightly from the hip and propel yourself quickly to an upright position. Slowly sit back down and, as soon as you touch the seat, repeat.

Power-stepping

The benefit of this exercise is that you can target all the muscles of your upper thighs and hips by varying the direction of your steps. Start by stepping from side to side, as described. As a variation, change the step to forward and back then try it on a diagonal.

Begin at Level 1 and progress at your own pace to Levels 2 & 3	
LEVEL 1	10 reps (1 rep = both sides), light band: 1–2 sets
LEVEL 2	12–15 reps, medium band: 1–2 sets
LEVEL 3	8–12 reps, heavy band: 2–3 sets

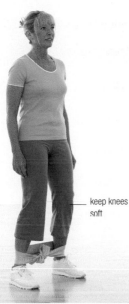

keep knees soft

2 Leading with the right leg, quickly step to the side then slowly (on a count of three) bring the left foot in toward the right, keeping tension in the band. Without touching your foot to the ground, quickly step to the left then bring the right foot in. Continue stepping from side to side.

feel it here

1 Tie the band into a loop (*see p32*), adjusting it so it is taut but not tight when you stand with your feet about hip-width apart. Rest your hands by your sides.

JOAN'S TIP

If you have any knee pain, try looping the band above your knees for this exercise.

Lunge/squat combo

Performing the front lunge and side squat in combination adds elements of balance, weight-shift, and change of direction into the strengthening formula. Begin by doing the sequence without weights then progress to holding a free weight in each hand (*see p35*).

Begin at Level 1 and progress at your own pace to Levels 2 & 3	
LEVEL 1	10 reps (1 rep = lunge/squat): 1 set
LEVEL 2	12–15 reps, holding 3–5lb weights: 1 set
LEVEL 3	8–12 reps, holding 8–10lb weights: 1 set

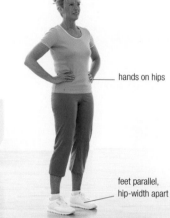

hands on hips

feet parallel, hip-width apart

keep torso upright

1 Stand with feet parallel, hip-width apart, hands resting on your hips (*inset*). Transfer your weight to the right leg and inhale as you step forward with your left leg, coming up on the ball of the right foot. Bend both knees so front knee is bent directly over ankle and back knee is lowered toward the floor.

knee directly over ankle

back knee lowered toward floor

JOAN'S TIP

Learn proper form by performing these exercises separately before combining them.

2 Pause in the lunge position then exhale and spring back to the starting position with feet parallel, hip-width apart, and hands on hips. Keep the knees soft.

3 Step to the side with the right leg. Keeping your weight evenly centered on both legs, inhale and bend your knees into a squatting position. On the exhale, straighten knees and step right leg back to center. Stepping forward with right leg, repeat combination sequence, stepping front and side with the right leg. Complete all reps then switch legs.

knees soft

feet parallel,
hip-width apart

forward lean
to torso

reach back
with your
hips

do not let
knees
collapse
inward

step to the right

Cross-body reach: beginner

Our ability to balance begins a subtle decline after the age of 40, the change occurring so slowly that we are usually unaware of it. There is also normally a marked difference between the left and right sides. With practice, however, you can minimize this imbalance.

Begin at Level 1 and progress at your own pace to Levels 2 & 3	
LEVEL 1	10 reps each side, holding chair: 1 set
LEVEL 2	10 reps, without holding chair: 1 set
LEVEL 3	10 reps, without holding chair, eyes closed: 1 set

1 Stand with all your weight on your left leg. Bend your right knee and raise the leg behind you, foot in the air. If necessary, hold on to the back of a chair to help you balance; otherwise relax your left arm by your side. Reach across your body with your right arm at shoulder level then return it to your side. Repeat as directed, keeping the foot off the ground. Switch sides and repeat.

arm raised to shoulder level

lightly hold chair for balance

keep knee soft

JOAN'S TIP

Always start with your less stable side, to give it mental as well as physical priority.

Cross-body reach: intermediate/advanced

The level of difficulty is increased here by altering your center of gravity as you bend forward to touch the weight. For a more advanced variation, pick the weight up with one or both hands and lift it to your chest. Come to an upright position, then return the weight to the floor.

Begin at Level 1 and progress at your own pace to Levels 2 & 3	
LEVEL 1	10 reps each side, touching weight: 1 set
LEVEL 2	10 reps, 3lb (1kg) weight: 1 set
LEVEL 3	10 reps, 5lb (2kg) weight: 1 set

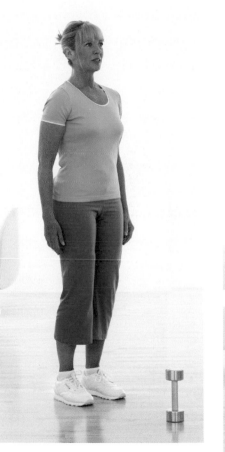

1 Stand with your feet parallel, hip-width apart. Position a free weight (or filled water bottle) upright on the floor at arm's length in front of the right leg. Arms are relaxed by your sides.

2 Balancing on the left leg, bend forward from the hip, reaching with your right arm to touch the free weight on the floor. Return to a fully upright position without allowing the left foot to touch the floor. Do all reps on one side, then switch sides and repeat.

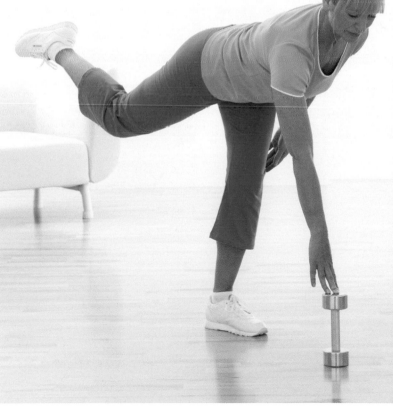

Calf raise/toe lift

The tibialis anterior (*see pp28–29*), in the front of the shin, performs the action of lifting the foot; it is the first muscle in the body to begin to lose strength and this can affect walking ability. This exercise strengthens it along with the major calf muscle, the gastrocnemius.

Begin at Level 1 and progress at your own pace to Levels 2 & 3	
LEVEL 1	10 reps: 1 set
LEVEL 2	15 reps: 1 set
LEVEL 3	20 reps: 1 set

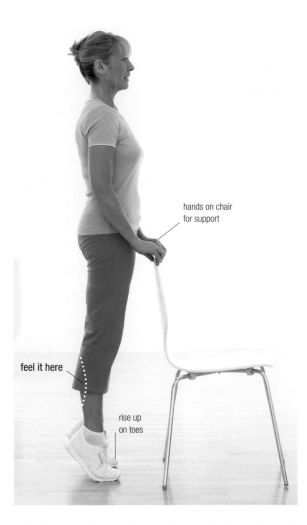

hands on chair for support

feel it here

rise up on toes

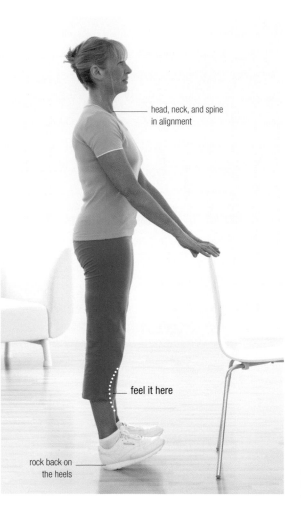

head, neck, and spine in alignment

feel it here

rock back on the heels

1 Stand behind a chair, with your feet parallel and hip-width apart. Rest your hands lightly on the back of the chair for support. Lift both heels off the floor as high as possible, so you are standing on your toes.

2 Lower your heels to the floor. Rock back onto the heels and lift both forefeet as high as you can, reaching the toes toward the ceiling. Repeat as directed, alternating the movements between calf raise and toe lift.

Lat pull-down

Training the latissimus dorsi (*see pp28–29*) will firm the sides of your back, improving your posture as well as your figure. Strengthening this powerful muscle will also enhance your ability to perform your daily activities with ease to maintain a young body age.

Begin at Level 1 and progress at your own pace to Levels 2 & 3	
LEVEL 1	10 reps, light band: 1–2 sets
LEVEL 2	12–15 reps, medium band: 1–2 sets
LEVEL 3	8–12 reps, heavy band: 2–3 sets

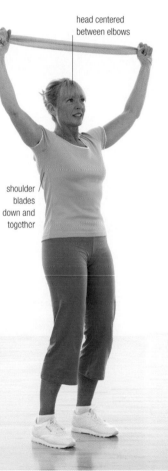

head centered between elbows

shoulder blades down and together

feel it here

2 Inhale, then as you exhale lower your arms out to the sides, stretching the band to the top of your chest. Hold for a second and then release. Keep the elbows rounded at a fixed angle as you slowly raise your arms overhead, returning to the starting position.

1 Holding the band, extend your arms overhead, palms facing forward and elbows slightly rounded. Put a little tension into the band.

Incline chest press

This exercise and the one opposite both build strength in the pectorals and the deltoid (*see pp28–29*)—the same muscles as are involved in push-ups. After eight weeks of doing these exercises, you should be able to perform more push-ups with less effort.

Begin at Level 1 and progress at your own pace to Levels 2 & 3	
LEVEL 1	10 reps, light band: 1–2 sets
LEVEL 2	12–15 reps, medium band: 1–2 sets
LEVEL 3	8–12 reps, heavy band: 2–3 sets

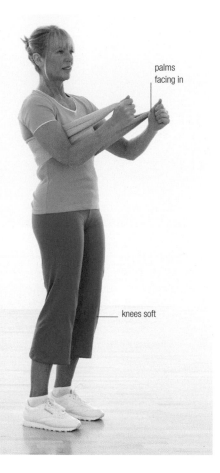

palms facing in

knees soft

extend arms upward at 45-degree angle

2 Exhale as you extend your arms upward at a 45-degree angle. Pause, then inhale and slowly return to the starting position. Remember to maintain tension in the band throughout the movement. Repeat for all reps.

1 Center band across the shoulder blades and adjust to its full width. Bending elbows close to your sides, hold your hands in front of your shoulders, pulling the band taut. Draw your shoulder blades down and together.

Shoulder flexion/extension

The shoulders provide a link between the large muscle groups of the back and chest. Strengthening them empowers all upper body movements, from those involved in household chores to sports skills. This exercise strengthens both the front and the back of the shoulder.

Begin at Level 1 and progress at your own pace to Levels 2 & 3	
LEVEL 1	10 reps, light band: 1–2 sets
LEVEL 2	12–15 reps, medium band: 1–2 sets
LEVEL 3	8–12 reps, heavy band: 2–3 sets

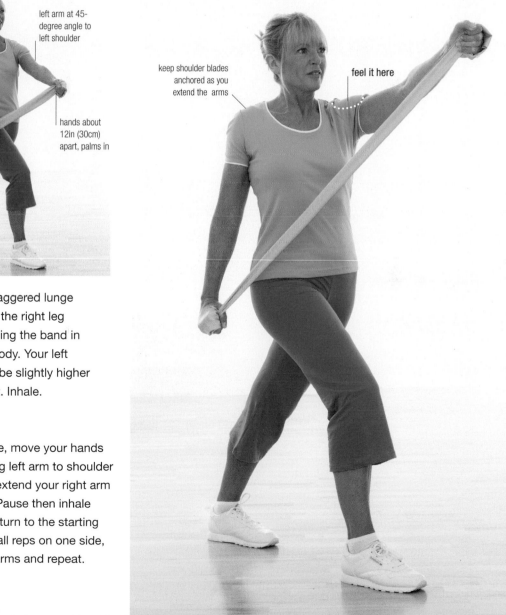

left arm at 45-degree angle to left shoulder

hands about 12in (30cm) apart, palms in

keep shoulder blades anchored as you extend the arms

feel it here

1 Stand in a staggered lunge position with the right leg forward, holding the band in front of the body. Your left hand should be slightly higher than the right. Inhale.

2 As you exhale, move your hands apart by lifting left arm to shoulder level as you extend your right arm behind you. Pause then inhale and slowly return to the starting position. Do all reps on one side, then switch arms and repeat.

Double biceps curl

A strong biceps makes it easier to lift and carry, whether it's a suitcase or roasting pan, a laptop or groceries. This is an upper body exercise and the legs are just anchoring the band, but it still makes sense to switch legs if you are doing more than one set.

Begin at Level 1 and progress at your own pace to Levels 2 & 3	
LEVEL 1	10 reps, light band: 1–2 sets
LEVEL 2	12–15 reps, medium band: 1–2 sets
LEVEL 3	8–12 reps, heavy band: 2–3 sets

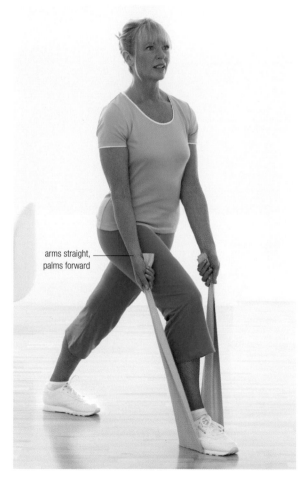

arms straight, palms forward

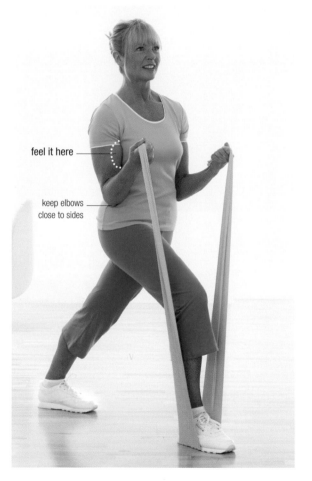

feel it here

keep elbows close to sides

1 Stand in a staggered lunge position with the right leg forward and the right knee bent over the ankle. Anchor the band securely under the right foot, holding the ends of the band with your arms straight, palms facing forward. Keep your wrists straight. Inhale.

2 As you exhale, bend your elbows, pulling the band up and in toward your shoulders. Hold for a moment, then slowly release. If the band is a little short for your height, loop it under your thigh instead of anchoring it with your foot. Repeat as directed.

Triceps push-down

This is another good exercise for firming and strengthening the upper arm, in this case the muscle at the back of the arm. To protect your neck from friction during the exercise, place a hand towel, folded lengthwise, around the back of your neck and center the band on it.

Begin at Level 1 and progress at your own pace to Levels 2 & 3	
LEVEL 1	10 reps, light band: 1–2 sets
LEVEL 2	12–15 reps, medium band: 1–2 sets
LEVEL 3	8–12 reps, heavy band: 2–3 sets

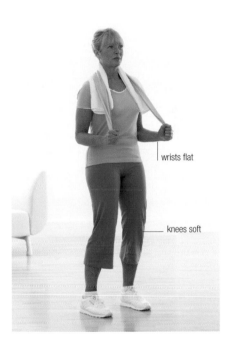

wrists flat

knees soft

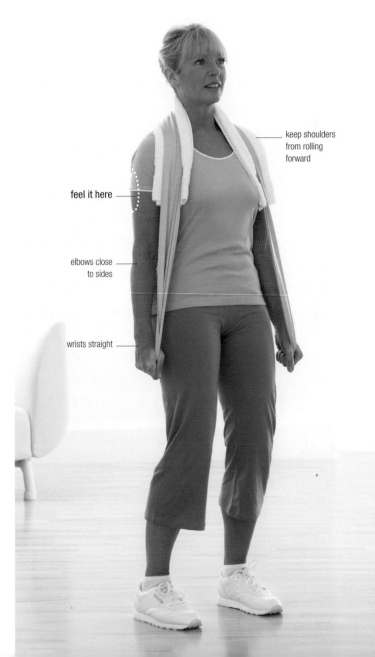

keep shoulders from rolling forward

feel it here

elbows close to sides

wrists straight

1 Holding the band as shown, draw your shoulder blades down and together. With your elbows bent at right angles, palms facing in, the band should be taut. Inhale.

2 As you exhale, straighten your arms toward the floor, being careful to keep your elbows close to your sides and your wrists straight. Do not allow your shoulders to roll forward. Repeat for the required number of reps.

Let-down

If you are just beginning to work your abdominals, or simply want to add some variety to your routine, try rolling down toward the floor instead of curling up as in the Basic crunch (*opposite*). Both exercises target the rectus abdominis muscle (*see pp28–29*).

Begin at Level 1 and progress at your own pace to Levels 2 & 3	
LEVEL 1	10 reps: 1–2 sets
LEVEL 2	15 reps: 1–2 sets
LEVEL 3	20 reps: 2–3 sets

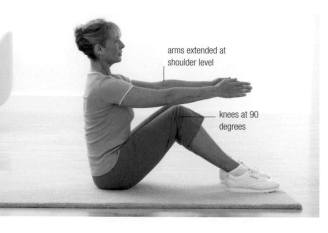

arms extended at shoulder level

knees at 90 degrees

1 Sit up straight on the floor, knees bent at 90 degrees, feet flat on the floor. Pull your torso as close as you can to your thighs and extend your arms to the front at shoulder level with the palms facing in. Inhale.

2 As you exhale, slowly roll down vertebra by vertebra, rounding your lower back, until you are about halfway down. Lift back up to the starting position. If you do not have the strength to lift back up, push off with your arms.

JOAN'S TIP

To increase the intensity, hold for 5–10 seconds before lifting up again.

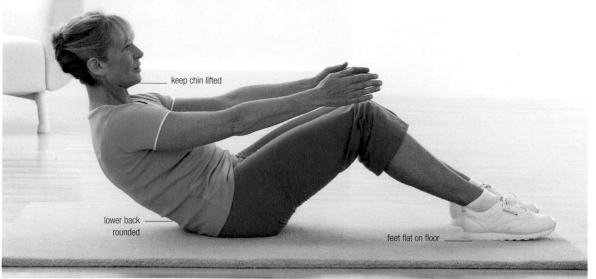

keep chin lifted

lower back rounded

feet flat on floor

Basic crunch

It takes focus and body awareness to perfect the execution of the basic crunch. The key is in the breathing and in abdominal compression: every time you lift your head and shoulders off the floor, exhale forcefully and pull the belly button in toward the spine.

Begin at Level 1 and progress at your own pace to Levels 2 & 3	
LEVEL 1	10 reps: 1–2 sets
LEVEL 2	15 reps: 1–2 sets
LEVEL 3	20 reps: 2–3 sets

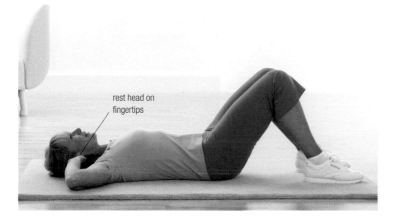

rest head on fingertips

1 Lie on your back on the floor, knees bent at 90 degrees, feet flat. To avoid pulling on your neck, place your fingertips behind your ears and rest your head lightly on them, elbows wide. Inhale.

2 As you exhale, pull your belly button in toward your spine and lift your head and shoulders 30 degrees off the floor. Keep your chin lifted. Pause at the top then inhale and lower your shoulder blades back to the floor.

Towel-assisted crunch
To bring your chest a little closer to your knees when lifting up, pull on a folded towel placed under your thighs. Hold for 5 seconds.

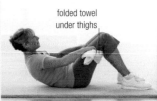

folded towel under thighs

chin lifted

pull belly button in toward spine

elbows wide

THE **46–55** WARM-UP

Step-ups are an efficient way to warm up and will also improve your performance on the Step test (*see p19*). The height of the platform, the speed of stepping, and the weight held determine the intensity of the work. After you learn the steps, try holding 3lb (1kg) weights and work up to 8lb (4kg) per hand, as long as you can maintain proper form.

Step-up

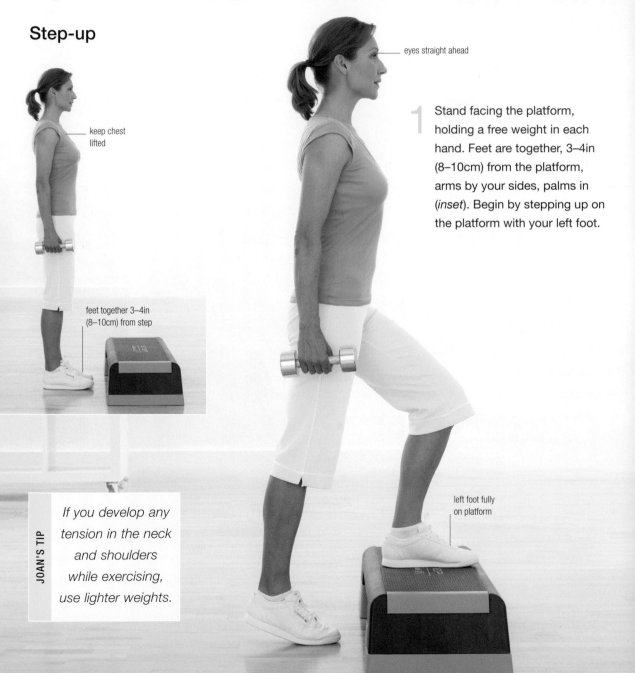

keep chest lifted

feet together 3–4in (8–10cm) from step

eyes straight ahead

1 Stand facing the platform, holding a free weight in each hand. Feet are together, 3–4in (8–10cm) from the platform, arms by your sides, palms in (*inset*). Begin by stepping up on the platform with your left foot.

left foot fully on platform

JOAN'S TIP

If you develop any tension in the neck and shoulders while exercising, use lighter weights.

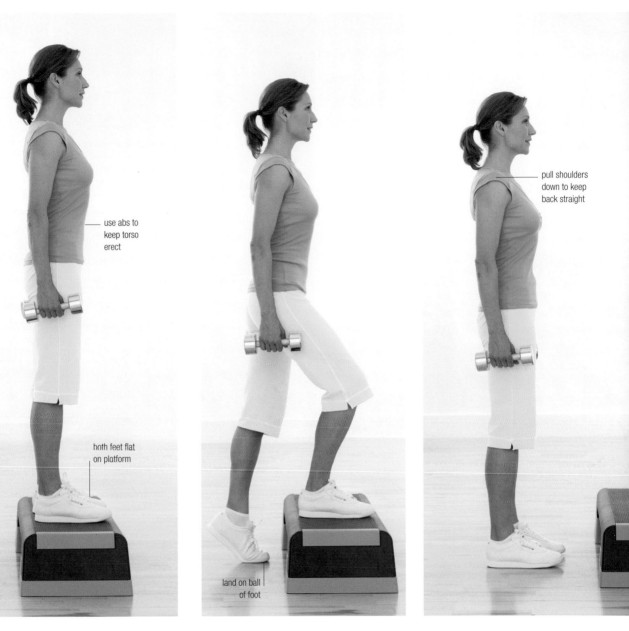

use abs to
keep torso
erect

pull shoulders
down to keep
back straight

both feet flat
on platform

land on ball
of foot

2 As soon as the left foot is
flat on the platform, step
up with the right foot so
both feet are on top. Arms
are straight, close to your
sides, and wrists straight.

3 Immediately step down with
your left leg, landing on the ball
of your foot and rolling down
through the heel. Keep your
head, neck, and spine aligned
as you step up and down.

4 Step down with your right
foot so both feet are back
on the floor. Continue
stepping rhythmically in
the pattern of "up, up,
down, down."
• **Reps** Do 20 step-ups, then
change lead foot and repeat

Step-up with alternating lead feet

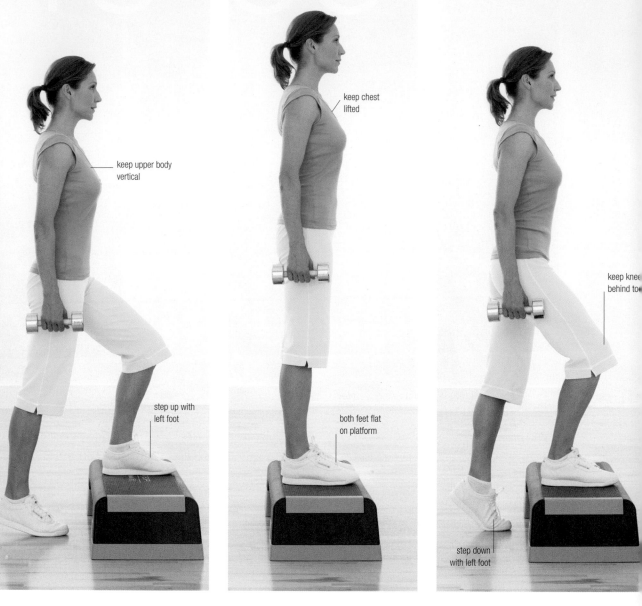

keep upper body vertical

step up with left foot

keep chest lifted

both feet flat on platform

keep knee behind to[

step down with left foot

1 Holding a free weight in each hand, stand facing the platform as before (*see p58*). Step onto the platform with the left foot.

2 As soon as the left foot is flat on the platform, step up with the right foot so both feet are on top. Keep your arms straight down by your sides.

3 Step down with your left leg, landing on the ball of your foot and rolling down through the heel.

Step-up with biceps curl

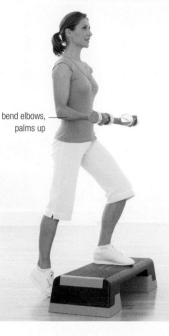

bend elbows,
palms up

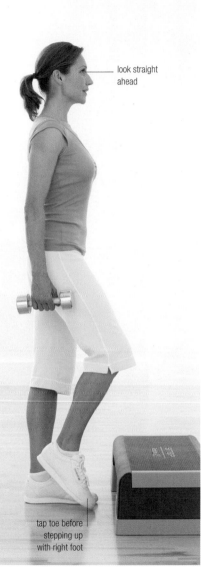

look straight
ahead

tap toe before
stepping up
with right foot

bring weights up
to shoulder level

both feet on
platform

1   Continue alternating step-ups, holding the weights with palms facing forward. As you step up with the left foot, start to bring the weights up toward your shoulders.

2   As you step up with the right foot, bring the weights up fully to shoulder level. Step down with the left foot, then tap with the right foot as you straighten your arms. Immediately step up with the right foot; continue, alternating sides.
 • **Reps** Do 20 reps

4   Step down with the right foot, tapping the toes on the floor before immediately stepping up again with the right foot. Continue stepping in this pattern of "up, up, down, change."
 • **Reps** Do 20 reps (one rep = both sides)

Straddle step

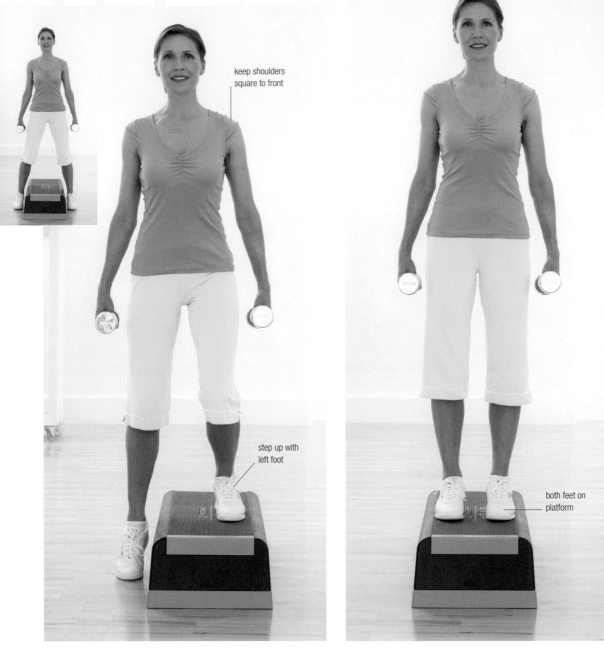

keep shoulders
square to front

step up with
left foot

both feet on
platform

1 Stand with one foot on either side of the platform, close to the step. Hold a free weight in each hand, palms facing in and wrists straight (*inset*). Keeping the knees soft, step up onto the platform with the left leg.

2 As soon as the left foot is flat on the platform, step up with the right foot, so both feet are centered on top of the step. Be aware of the distribution of your body weight so that you stay balanced on both legs.

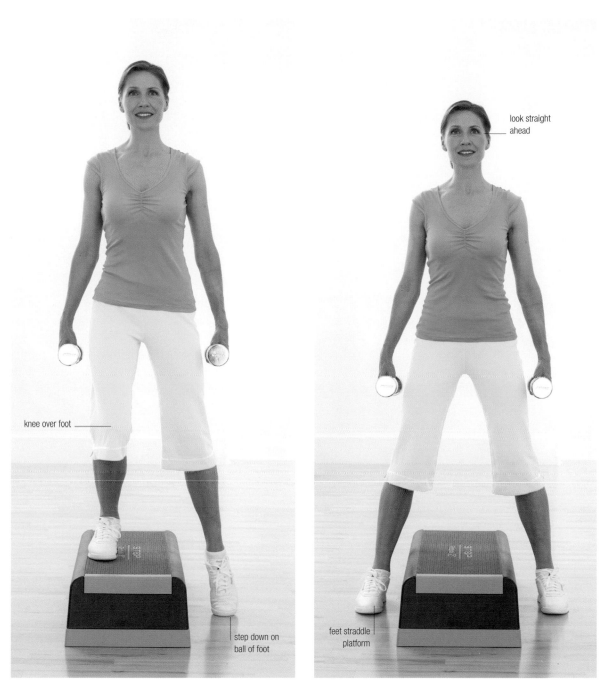

knee over foot

look straight
ahead

step down on
ball of foot

feet straddle
platform

3 Maintaining the same rhythm as in the
previous step-ups (pp58–61), step down
with the left foot to the side of the platform,
landing on the ball of your foot and rolling
down through the heel.

4 Immediately step down with the right foot,
so that you are back in the starting position,
straddling the step. Continue stepping in this
pattern of "up, up, down, down."
• **Reps** Do 20 reps then change lead foot and repeat

Over the top

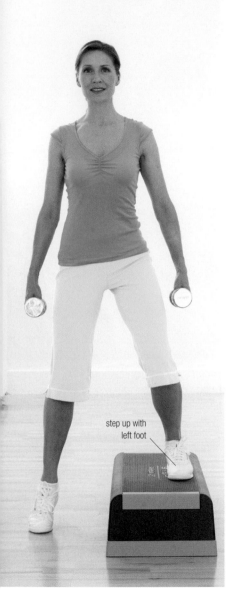

keep ribs
over hips

soft
knees

step up with
left foot

both feet on
platform

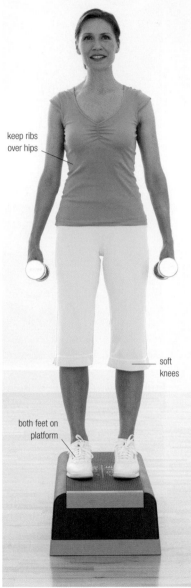

look straight
ahead

step down and tap
with right foot

1 Stand with your left side
to the platform, feet
parallel, about 4in (10cm)
from the step. Holding a
free weight in each hand,
palms in, step up onto the
platform with the left foot.

2 As soon as the left foot is flat
on the platform, step up with
your right foot, so both feet
are centered on the step,
about 4in (10cm) apart.
Hands are straight down by
your sides, palms facing in.

3 Step down to the other side
of the platform with left foot
and tap with the right. Step
up with the right foot and
move across to other side.
• **Reps** Do 20 reps (one rep =
both sides)

THE **46–55** PROGRAM

You can work through these exercises in the order they are presented, or, to vary your routine, intersperse the warm-up exercises (*see pp58–64*) with the resistance exercises to create a circuit-training workout. Keeping your heart rate elevated during the session will benefit your cardiovascular system while strengthening your muscles and bones.

Balance clock

This exercise has several benefits: every time you lower yourself toward the floor, you are doing a mini-squat that works the entire leg, from hip to ankle. Working one leg at a time helps you spot any asymmetries in strength and balance, so you can focus on even development.

Begin at Level 1 and progress at your own pace to Levels 2 & 3	
LEVEL 1	3 reps in each position: 1 set
LEVEL 2	5 reps in each position: 1 set
LEVEL 3	10 reps in each position: 1 set

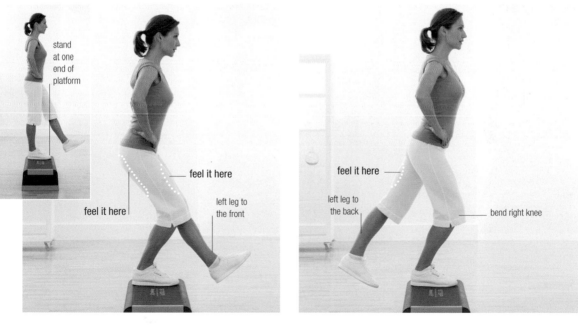

stand at one end of platform

feel it here

feel it here

left leg to the front

feel it here

left leg to the back

bend right knee

1 Stand on right leg on a 6–10in- (15–25cm-) high step. Extend left leg forward to 12 o'clock (*inset*). Bend the right knee and slowly lower the left leg. Push through the heel of the right leg to straighten up to the starting position.

2 Keeping the hips facing forward throughout, continue around the clock, extending your leg out to the side (9 o'clock) and then to the back (6 o'clock), repeating the squats three times at each position. Repeat with the other leg.

Side squat with weights

This is a great exercise for shaping the glutes in the buttocks (*see pp28–29*). Anytime you step up onto a platform, climb stairs, or hike up an incline, you are giving these muscles a lift. As an added health benefit, you are also strengthening the femur (thigh bone).

Begin at Level 1 and progress at your own pace to Levels 2 & 3	
LEVEL 1	10 reps, without weights: 1–2 sets
LEVEL 2	12–15 reps, holding 3–5lb (1–2kg) weights: 1–2 sets
LEVEL 3	8–12 reps, holding 8–10lb (4–5kg) weights; 2–3 sets

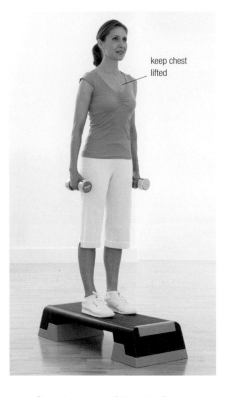

keep chest lifted

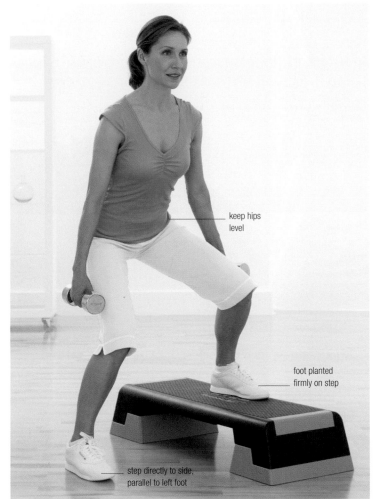

keep hips level

foot planted firmly on step

step directly to side, parallel to left foot

1 Stand on top of the platform, facing one end. The feet are parallel, hip-width apart. Hold a free weight in each hand, palms facing in. If you prefer, you can bend your elbows and hold one weight on each shoulder, or rest them on your hips (*see p68*).

2 Step off the platform with the right leg. Inhale as you slowly bend both knees into a full squat. Exhale, contract the glutes, and push through the left leg to return to the starting position. Repeat as directed, then switch sides and repeat.

Knee-up with overhead reach

This exercise requires the coordination of several muscle groups working together. The large leg muscles are synchronized with those of the shoulders and upper back and at the same time the core muscles are engaged as the abdominals and spinal extensors work as stabilizers.

Begin at Level 1 and progress at your own pace to Levels 2 & 3	
LEVEL 1	10 reps, holding one 3lb (1kg) weight: 1 set
LEVEL 2	12–15 reps, holding one 5lb (2kg) weight: 1 set
LEVEL 3	8–12 reps, holding one 8lb (4kg) weight: 1 set

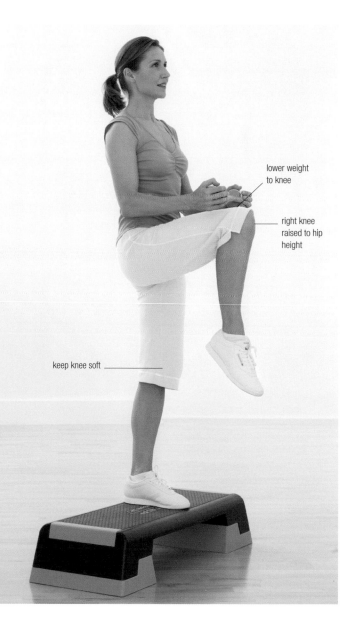

feel it here

arms above shoulder level

knee bent, over ankle

roll onto ball of foot

lower weight to knee

right knee raised to hip height

keep knee soft

1 Plant the left foot fully on the step. Holding a free weight with both hands as shown, extend your arms in front of you on a diagonal, above shoulder level.

2 Bring right knee up to hip height as you bend your arms and touch the weight to your knee. Return to the starting position. Repeat as directed, switch sides, and repeat.

Lunge and narrow squat

The combination lunge and squat is an efficient way to overload the muscles of the glutes and thighs for firming and strengthening. Lunging onto the step is easier than lunging onto the floor. However, holding weights and adding the squat increases the intensity.

Begin at Level 1 and progress at your own pace to Levels 2 & 3	
LEVEL 1	10 reps (1 rep = both sides), no weights, 1 set
LEVEL 2	12–15 reps, holding 3–5lb (1–2kg) weights: 1 set
LEVEL 3	8–12 reps, holding 8–10lb (4–5kg) weights: 1 set

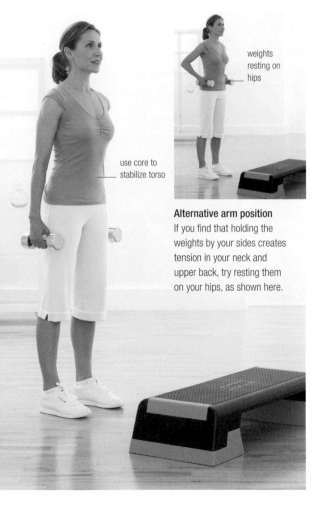

use core to stabilize torso

weights resting on hips

Alternative arm position
If you find that holding the weights by your sides creates tension in your neck and upper back, try resting them on your hips, as shown here.

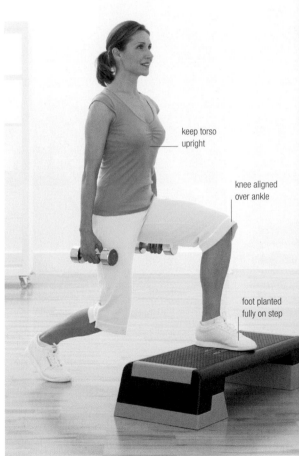

keep torso upright

knee aligned over ankle

foot planted fully on step

1 Stand facing the length of the platform, about 18in (46cm) away from it. The feet are parallel and hip-width apart. Hold a free weight in each hand with your arms straight by your sides, palms facing in. Keep the knees soft.

2 Lunge onto the step with your left foot, making sure it is planted fully on the platform. Keep your left knee aligned over the ankle. Bend both knees in a lunge, coming up on the toes of your right foot. Arms are straight by your sides.

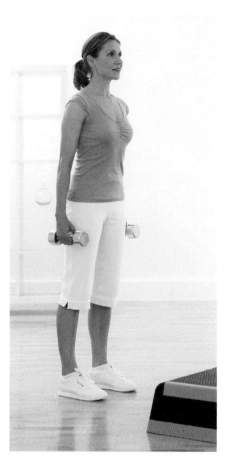

3 Straighten both legs as you spring back with your left leg to the starting position. Feet are parallel and hip-width apart, and arms by your sides, palms in.

4 Bend both knees in a squat. Return to the starting position and repeat, lunging with the right leg. (This completes one rep.) Continue alternating lead legs as you lunge, interspersing one narrow squat between each set of left and right leg lunges. Repeat as directed.

torso leaning forward

spine straight

bend knees in narrow squat

Calf raise

The step provides a perfect opportunity for performing a calf raise with an increased range of motion, which works the muscle throughout its entire length. If you don't have a step, you can obtain the same advantage by working off any raised step or curb.

Begin at Level 1 and progress at your own pace to Levels 2 & 3	
LEVEL 1	10 reps each leg + 10 reps both legs: 1 set
LEVEL 2	15 reps each leg + 15 reps both legs: 1 set
LEVEL 3	20 reps each leg + 20 reps both legs: 1 set

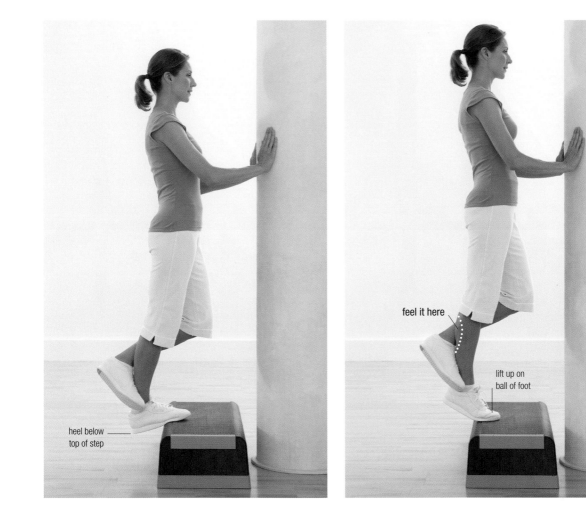

heel below top of step

feel it here

lift up on ball of foot

1 Stand with the ball of the right foot on the step, lightly holding a wall or chair for support. Hook your left foot around the right ankle to consolidate your body weight on the right side. Lower the right heel below the surface of the platform.

2 Exhale as you lift up on ball of right foot, then slowly lower heel below step surface. Repeat as directed, then switch sides. Finish with one set of both feet lifting up and dropping down together. Hang your heels off step to stretch.

One arm row

Many of us tend to neglect the important muscles of the back because they are out of view. However, back pain is a serious problem and affects millions in the work place. Strengthening the latissimus dorsi (*see pp28–29*) reduces the risk of back problems.

Begin at Level 1 and progress at your own pace to Levels 2 & 3	
LEVEL 1	10 reps, holding 5lb (2kg) weight: 1–2 sets
LEVEL 2	12–15 reps, 8lb (4kg) weight: 1–2 sets
LEVEL 3	8–12 reps, 10–12lb (5–5.5kg) weight: 2–3 sets

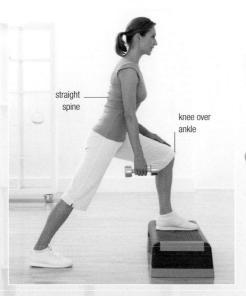

straight spine

knee over ankle

keep shoulder blade drawn back

feel it here

2 Draw the shoulder blade in toward the spine and hold it there during the entire exercise. Exhale as you bend your elbow, drawing the weight up to waist level. Inhale as you slowly return to starting position. Repeat as directed, then switch sides and repeat.

Stand in a staggered lunge position with your left foot on the step. Bend forward at the hip and place your left hand on your thigh. Hold one free weight in your right hand, palm facing in.

foot firmly planted on step

Front and side shoulder raise

This exercise works the front and middle aspects of the deltoid muscle (see pp28–29), which covers the top of the shoulder, providing natural "shoulder pads." Giving shape to this muscle improves the way you look in both sleeveless tops and jackets.

Begin at Level 1 and progress at your own pace to Levels 2 & 3	
LEVEL 1	10 reps, holding 2–3lb (0.5–1kg) weights: 1 set
LEVEL 2	12–15 reps, holding 5lb (2kg) weights: 1 set
LEVEL 3	8–12 reps, holding 8lb (4kg) weights: 1 set

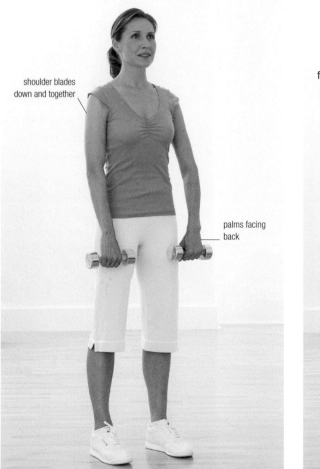

shoulder blades down and together

palms facing back

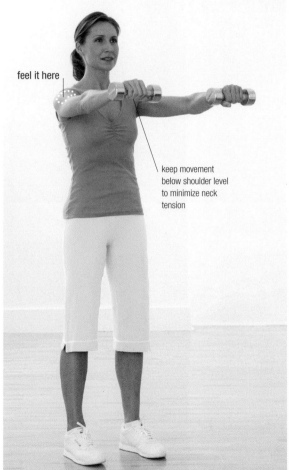

feel it here

keep movement below shoulder level to minimize neck tension

1 Stand with your feet parallel, hip-width apart, knees soft. Hold a free weight in each hand, arms in front of your thighs, palms facing back. Pull your shoulder blades down and together.

2 Breathe in then, as you exhale, lift both arms to the front, to shoulder height. Keep your wrists flat and your forearms parallel. Your arms should be straight but not stiff.

feel it here

feel it here

elbows rounded

palms down

shoulders back

palms facing in

4 Inhale, then, as you exhale, lift your arms out to the sides, to shoulder level (no higher), with your elbows in line with your shoulders. Keep your elbows slightly rounded, with palms facing down at the top of the movement. Inhale and slowly return to the starting position. Repeat the whole sequence as directed.

3 Pause for a moment, then slowly lower your arms to the starting position, keeping your shoulders back. Turn your arms, so that your palms now face in.

JOAN'S TIP

To isolate the shoulder properly, lead with your elbows, letting the forearms follow.

Modified push-up

Both the push-up and the chest fly (*opposite*) strengthen the pectoral and deltoid muscles (*see pp28–29*). Doing them on the step is a good way to begin building up strength, since the reduced range of motion makes this version easier than doing them on the floor.

Begin at Level 1 and progress at your own pace to Levels 2 & 3	
LEVEL 1	10 reps: 1–2 sets
LEVEL 2	12–15 reps: 1–2 sets
LEVEL 3	20 reps: 1–2 sets

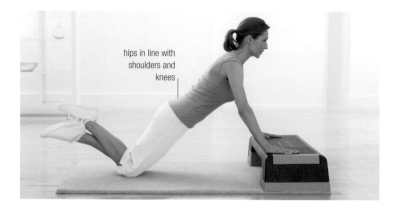

hips in line with shoulders and knees

1 Kneel in front of the step with your hands 3–4in (8–10cm) wider than chest-width apart. Drop your hips to form a straight line from shoulders to knees. Pull your abs tight to prevent your back from sagging and shift your weight forward of your knee caps to avoid direct pressure on them.

2 Draw your shoulder blades down and together and inhale as you bend your elbows out to the sides at right angles, lowering your chest toward the step. Exhale as you straighten your arms back to the starting position. Repeat the push-ups as directed.

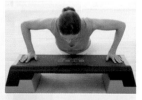

Bend your elbows out to the sides at 90 degrees as you lower your chest.

keep weight in front of knee caps

Advanced push-up
To increase the intensity, put your feet on the step and shift more body weight to the chest and shoulders.

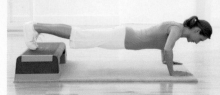

Chest fly

Some of my clients simply do not like push-ups, so we find alternatives such as the Chest fly, which work the same muscles. Building strength helps firm up the bustline and shape the front of the shoulder—as well as making the push-ups easier and not so objectionable.

Begin at Level 1 and progress at your own pace to Levels 2 & 3	
LEVEL 1	10 reps, holding 3lb (1kg) weights: 1–2 sets
LEVEL 2	12–15 reps, holding 5lb (2kg) weights: 1–2 sets
LEVEL 3	8–12 reps, holding 8–10lb (4–5kg) weights: 2–3 sets

palms in

elbows rounded

1 Lie on the step with your feet on the floor. Contract your abs to maintain neutral spine alignment and prevent the lower back from arching. Holding a free weight in each hand, palms in, extend your arms above your chest.

JOAN'S TIP

Keep your shoulder blades drawn down and together as you move your arms.

2 Anchor your shoulder blades, inhale, then slowly open your arms out to the sides in an arc motion. Exhale as you return to the starting position through the same arc, until the weights touch lightly at the top. Repeat the movements as directed.

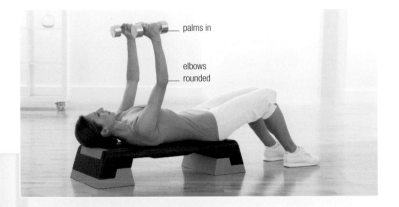

feel it here

shoulder blades anchored

elbows rounded

Triceps dip

When performing triceps dips, it is important to brace your shoulders properly to prevent them from rounding forward and straining the shoulder joint. If you have the right form, you will feel the triceps and the muscles between the shoulder blades working.

Begin at Level 1 and progress at your own pace to Levels 2 & 3	
LEVEL 1	10 reps: 1–2 sets
LEVEL 2	12–15 reps: 1–2 sets
LEVEL 3	20 reps: 1–2 sets

bend elbows behind you

do not let shoulders roll forward

lower hips toward floor

1 Sit on the edge of the step with knees bent, feet flat on the floor, arms straight, hands on edge of step. Supporting your weight with your arms, lift your hips off the step. Inhale and slowly bend your elbows, lowering your hips toward the floor.

Straight leg variation
To increase the intensity of the triceps dip, straighten your legs in front of you before dipping down. This shifts more of your body's weight onto your upper body, adding resistance.

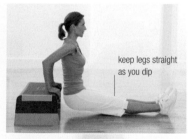

keep legs straight as you dip

2 As you exhale, press through the palms to straighten your arms, lifting your hips back up to the level of the platform. Be careful not to lock the elbows. Repeat as directed.

feel it here

straighten arms to raise hips

press through palms

Bicycle crunch

Studies have shown this to be one of the most effective abdominal exercises because it works all four of the muscles of the abdomen: the rectus abdominis, the internal and external obliques, and the transversus abdominis (*see pp28–29*).

Begin at Level 1 and progress at your own pace to Levels 2 & 3	
LEVEL 1	10 reps (1 rep = both sides): 1–2 sets
LEVEL 2	12–15 reps: 1–2 sets
LEVEL 3	20 reps: 1–2 sets

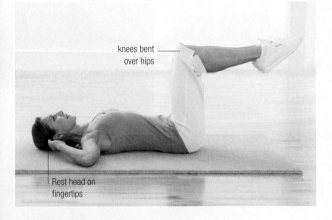

knees bent over hips

Rest head on fingertips

1 Lie on your back with your knees bent over your hips, calves parallel to the floor, feet in the air. Rest your head lightly on your fingertips, thumbs by your ears.

JOAN'S TIP

To intensify the work of the Bicycle crunch, hold each twist for three seconds.

2 Tighten your abs and lift your head and shoulders off the floor, twisting the left shoulder toward the right knee as you extend the left leg. Return to the start position and repeat on the other side. Exhale with every lift and twist. Repeat as directed.

lift head and shoulders

keep elbow wide

feel it here

extend leg at 45-degree angle

feel it here

Dead bug

Both this exercise and the one opposite work the abdominal muscles without flexing the spine. As well as adding variety to a program of crunches, they offer a safe way to target the abdominals if you have a spinal condition such as osteoporosis.

Begin at Level 1 and progress at your own pace to Levels 2 & 3	
LEVEL 1	5–10 reps (1 rep = both sides): 1 set
LEVEL 2	15 reps: 1 set
LEVEL 3	10 reps, holding extended position 5–10 secs: 1 set

hands directly over shoulders

hips and knees at right angles

1 Lie on your back with your hips and knees bent at right angles, feet in the air. Extend your arms up toward the ceiling, directly over your shoulders, palms facing inward.

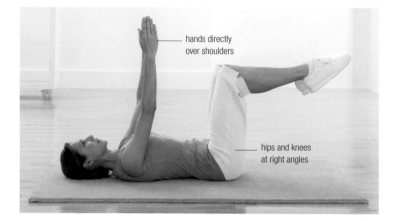

2 Draw your belly button toward your spine. Lower your left arm overhead as you slowly straighten the right leg, lowering it as far as possible without arching your back. Bring the left knee in closer to your chest. Return to the start position and repeat, alternating sides.

left knee in toward chest

left arm lowered overhead

feel it here

right leg lowered toward floor

do not arch lower back

Plank with knee bend

As well as working the abdominal muscles, this exercise offers the added benefit of engaging the spinal extensors (*see pp28–29*) for well-rounded core training and back strengthening. Keep your abdominals engaged to stabilize your torso throughout the exercise.

Begin at Level 1 and progress at your own pace to Levels 2 & 3	
LEVEL 1	5–10 reps (1 rep = both sides): 1–2 sets
LEVEL 2	12–15 reps; 1–2 sets
LEVEL 3	20 reps: 1–2 sets

1 In the start position (*inset*) tighten your abs to stabilize your torso. Extend your legs, coming up on the toes to create a straight line from head to heels. Squeeze the shoulder blades down and together.

straight line from head to heels

hands under shoulders, palms forward

2 Keeping your hips square to the floor and the torso stabilized, lower your right knee close to the floor, then straighten it and switch legs. Continue alternating sides to complete the set as directed.

shoulder blades down and together

keep hips level

right knee lowered toward floor

THE **36-45** WARM-UP

Bouncing on the stability ball will get your heart pumping and your blood flowing. Begin to bounce by pushing your feet into the floor and tightening your hips and thighs to lift your body weight off the ball. Your abdominals and spinal extensors (*see pp28–29*) will engage simultaneously to keep your torso upright as you challenge your balance and coordination.

Bounce into full march

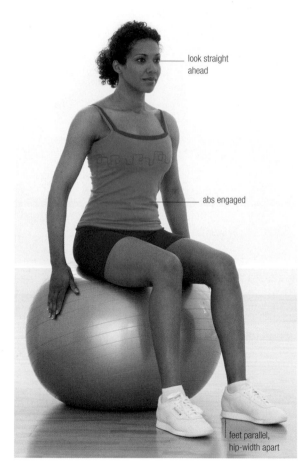

look straight ahead

abs engaged

feet parallel, hip-width apart

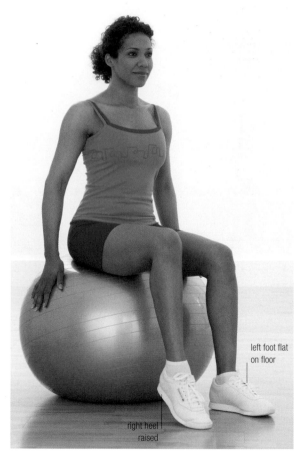

left foot flat on floor

right heel raised

1 Sit up tall on the ball, slightly forward of the center. Feet are parallel, hip-width apart, arms down by your sides. Lightly touch your hands on either side of the ball for balance. Keep your upper body vertical, look straight ahead, and pull your abs in toward your belly button.

2 Begin bouncing. When you have established a steady rhythm and feel balanced on the ball, push the toes of your right foot into the floor, raising your heel. With the next bounce, switch sides, raising the heel of the left foot. Continue alternating sides with each bounce.

3 As you continue bouncing, lift your right foot off the floor and raise your right knee; the left foot remains on the floor. On the next bounce, raise the left foot off the floor and raise your left knee. Continue alternating sides, as if marching. Arms remain by your sides

right knee raised

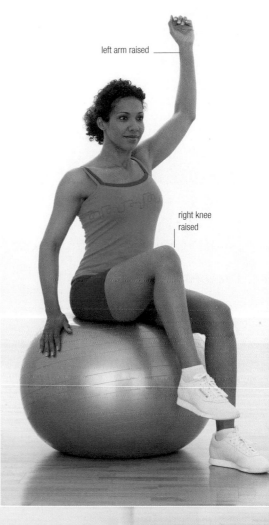

left arm raised

right knee raised

4 Now add upper body movement by raising the opposite arm with each knee lift. Gradually reach higher, straightening the arm toward the ceiling. Continue alternating sides.

• **Reps** Do 20 reps (one rep = both sides)

Kick-out with arm raise

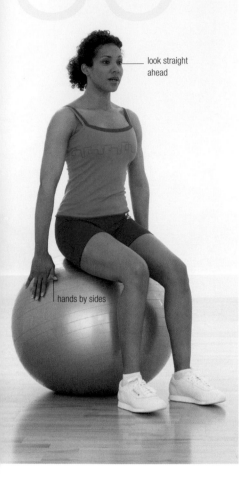

look straight
ahead

hands by sides

2 On one bounce, extend your right leg forward and slightly out to the side, landing on your heel with your toe lifted. At the same time raise your left arm up and slightly to the side. On the next bounce, return to center; repeat, alternating sides.

• **Reps** Do 20 reps (one rep = both sides)

left arm raised
and to the side

1 In this transition phase, continue to bounce with your arms down by your sides, hands touching the ball or gently swinging.

right leg
extended

Cossack dance

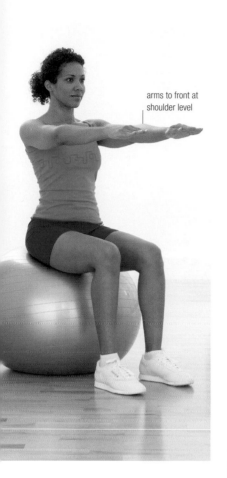

arms to front at
shoulder level

2 With one bounce, extend the right leg and right arm
out to the side and bring the left hand in front of the
shoulder. Keep the elbow out to the side at shoulder
level. With the next bounce return to the starting
position and repeat to the other side.

• **Reps** Do 20 reps (one rep = both sides)

right arm
out to side

left elbow bent, at
shoulder level

right leg extended
to side

1 In this transition to the next
movement, raise both arms
to the front at shoulder level
as you continue to bounce.
Palms are down and feet flat
on the floor, hip-width apart.

Jumping Jack

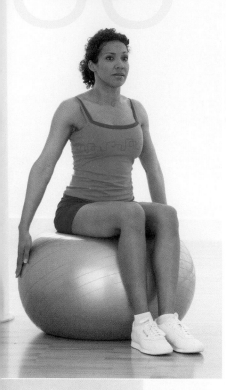

JOAN'S TIP

Jumping both feet apart in this exercise requires more control than keeping one foot on the ground.

2 With one bounce, jump the knees and feet apart, simultaneously raising the arms overhead. On the next bounce, jump the legs back to the starting position and bring your arms down, clapping the hands on the sides of the ball.
• **Reps** Do 20 reps

1 During the transition phase, continue to bounce with your arms by your sides, feet parallel and hip-width apart, preparing yourself for the movement.

THE **36–45** PROGRAM

As early as age 25, you may begin to experience subtle changes in your body composition that are not reflected in your scale weight. Even if you maintain your weight perfectly over time you can expect to lose about 5lb (2kg) of muscle and gain 5lb (2kg) of fat by age 50 unless you do resistance training, which defends against these changes.

Ball squat

This is a classic exercise using a stability ball. If you have never done squats, it is the perfect rehearsal for the free-standing version. Ball squats build strength in your legs and help you to learn proper alignment, keeping your knees over your ankles.

Begin at Level 1 and progress at your own pace to Levels 2 & 3	
LEVEL 1	10 reps, no weights: 1–2 sets
LEVEL 2	12–15 reps, holding 5–8lb (2–4kg) weights: 1–2 sets
LEVEL 3	8–12 reps, 10–12lb (5–5.5kg) weights: 2–3 sets

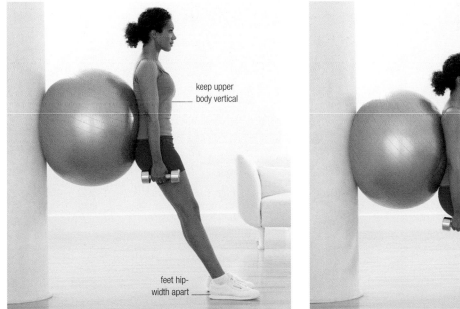

keep upper body vertical

feet hip-width apart

knees over ankles

1 Hold a free weight in each hand, palms facing in. Position the stability ball against the wall so it fits snugly in the natural curve of your spine. Leaning your weight against the ball, walk your feet forward until your legs are almost straight.

2 Keeping your back straight, slowly bend your knees until your thighs are parallel to the floor, or as far as you can go. Make sure your knees are directly over your ankles. Pause briefly, then tighten your buttocks to push back up.

Front lunge with ball

This lunge variation combines upper, lower, and core body movement, with all the muscles of the body working together. Exercises such as this, which simulate the way the body moves in daily life, prepare us to meet the demands of our lifestyle.

Begin at Level 1 and progress at your own pace to Levels 2 & 3	
LEVEL 1	10 reps: 1–2 sets
LEVEL 2	12–15 reps: 1–2 sets
LEVEL 3	20 reps: 1–2 sets

elbows bent at
right angles

feet parallel,
hip-width apart

1 Standing with your feet parallel, hip-width apart, hold the ball in front of your waist with both hands, elbows bent at right angles. Straighten your spine and tighten your abs.

2 Inhale as you step forward on the right leg. Bending both knees, reach forward and touch the ball to the floor. As you exhale, spring back to the starting position. Repeat as directed, then switch legs and repeat.

straight
spine

straight arms

come up on toes
of back foot

Side squat with knee lift

As well as shaping, toning, and strengthening the muscles of your hips, thighs, and buttocks, this exercise will challenge your balance, particularly if you pause with your knee up in step 2. Determine which leg needs more work on balance and begin with that side.

Begin at Level 1 and progress at your own pace to Levels 2 & 3	
LEVEL 1	10 reps: 1–2 sets
LEVEL 2	12–15 reps: 1–2 sets
LEVEL 3	20 reps: 1–2 sets

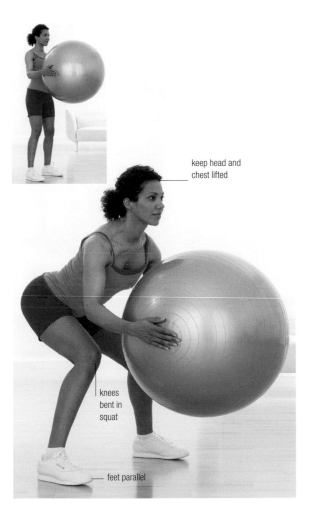

keep head and chest lifted

knees bent in squat

feet parallel

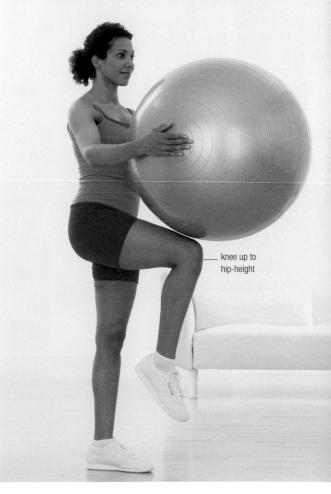

2 Exhale, straighten your legs, then bring the right knee up to hip height, touching the ball; immediately return to the squat position. Repeat as directed, then switch legs and repeat.

knee up to hip-height

1 Stand tall, feet parallel, hip-width apart, knees soft, holding the ball in front of you (*inset*). Take a wide step to the side with the right leg, keeping the feet parallel. Inhale and bend both knees to lower your hips into a squat.

Back leg lift on ball

This variation of a back leg lift targets three typical problem areas: the glutes, hamstrings, and inner thighs (*see pp28–29*). Doing it on the ball challenges your balance and stability, engaging the core muscles as your abdominals and back contract to maintain the position.

Begin at Level 1 and progress at your own pace to Levels 2 & 3	
LEVEL 1	10 reps: 1–2 sets
LEVEL 2	12–15 reps: 1–2 sets
LEVEL 3	20 reps: 1–2 sets

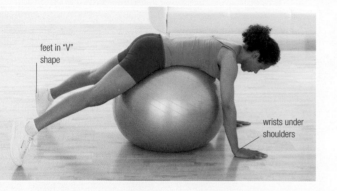

feet in "V" shape

wrists under shoulders

1 Lie over the ball and walk forward until your hips are resting on top of the ball. Arms are straight with wrists under your shoulders and your legs are extended, toes touching the floor. Separate your legs into a wide "V" shape.

2 Tighten your glutes and slowly raise your legs to hip height. Use your inner thighs to draw your legs together at the top. Pause, then slowly return your legs to a "V" shape on the floor. Repeat the movements as directed.

feet together

feel it here

head and neck aligned with spine

JOAN'S TIP

To maintain proper alignment of your head, neck, and spine, keep your nose down toward the floor.

Seated lat row

Training the latissimus dorsi (*see pp28–29*) will improve your performance in sports, putting more muscle into your tennis serve, golf swing, and swim stroke. If you are a runner it will reinforce your posture against the tendency to hunch the upper body.

Begin at Level 1 and progress at your own pace to Levels 2 & 3	
LEVEL 1	10 reps, holding 5lb (2kg) weights: 1–2 sets
LEVEL 2	12–15 reps, holding 8lb (4kg) weights: 1–2 sets
LEVEL 3	8–12 reps, 10–12lb (5–5.5kg) weights: 2–3 sets

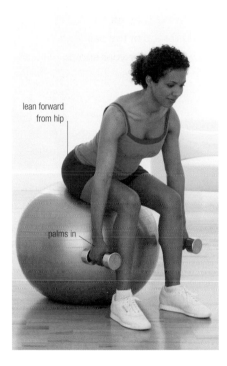

lean forward from hip

palms in

1 Sit on the ball, holding a free weight in each hand. Keeping your back straight, lean forward from the hip at a 45-degree angle. Draw your shoulder blades in toward your spine and inhale.

2 As you exhale, lift the weights up to your waist by bending your elbows behind you to shoulder level. Inhale as you slowly return to the starting position. Repeat as directed.

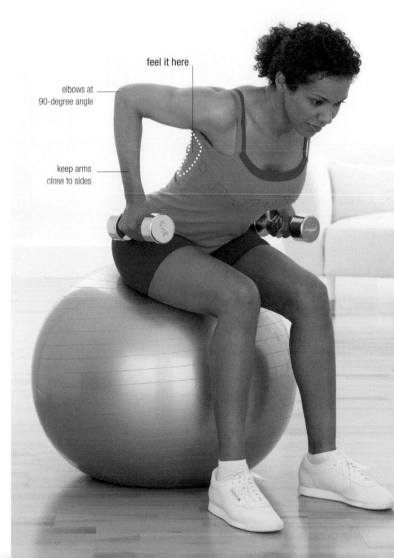

feel it here

elbows at 90-degree angle

keep arms close to sides

Pullover

This "feel-good" exercise gives a nice stretch to the abdomen while working the lats and pectoral muscles together, providing a smooth transition from back to chest work. To ensure that you target the proper muscles, keep your elbows rounded and move from the shoulder.

Begin at Level 1 and progress at your own pace to Levels 2 & 3	
LEVEL 1	10 reps, holding 3lb (1kg) weights: 1–2 sets
LEVEL 2	12–15 reps, holding 5lb (2kg) weights: 1–2 sets
LEVEL 3	8–12 reps, 8–10lb (4–5kg) weights: 2–3 sets

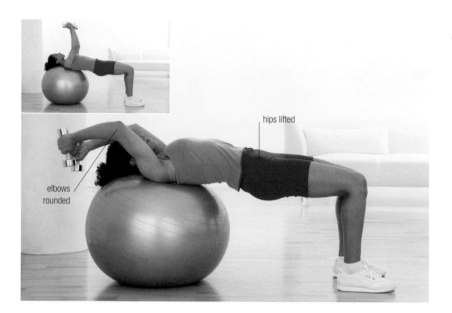

hips lifted

elbows rounded

1 Sit on the ball then roll forward until you are in bridge position, with the head, neck, and shoulders supported. Holding a weight in each hand, extend your arms to the ceiling, palms facing in (*inset*). Pull the shoulder blades down and together, inhale, then lower the weights overhead. Keep the arms shoulder-width apart, elbows rounded.

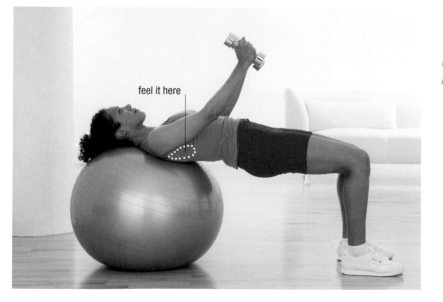

feel it here

2 As you exhale, pull the weights down over your chest to just above your waist. To make this exercise easier, you can rest the weights lightly together or hold just one larger weight with both hands. Keeping your hips lifted, repeat the movements as directed.

Alternating chest press

Here we take a classic exercise and make it more interesting by doing it on an unstable surface; this requires core stability and lower body strength to maintain the position. Perform the action one arm at a time to further challenge your torso stabilization.

Begin at Level 1 and progress at your own pace to Levels 2 & 3	
LEVEL 1	10 reps, holding 3lb (1kg) weights: 1–2 sets
LEVEL 2	12–15 reps, holding 5lb (2kg) weights: 1–2 sets
LEVEL 3	8–12 reps, holding 8–10lb (4–5kg) weights: 2–3 sets

1 From a seated position on the ball, and holding a free weight in each hand, roll down into bridge position. Extend your arms to the ceiling, then lower your elbows to your sides until they are bent at right angles.

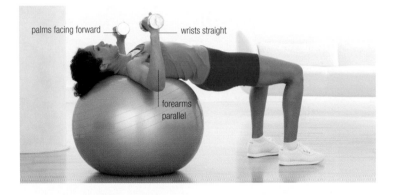

palms facing forward

wrists straight

forearms parallel

2 As you exhale, straighten one arm to the ceiling without locking the elbow. Inhale as you lower the weight to the starting position, pause, then repeat with the opposite arm. Alternate arms as you perform your repetitions.

arm straight but not stiff

feel it here

hips lifted

feet parallel, hip-width apart

Triceps extension

This muscle is a common trouble-spot for women, lying under the upper arm where fat tends to deposit. A two-part strategy for improving the shape and tone of the area is to firm up the muscle with weight-training and reduce the overlying fat with cardio work.

Begin at Level 1 and progress at your own pace to Levels 2 & 3	
LEVEL 1	10 reps, holding 3lb (1kg) weights: 1–2 sets
LEVEL 2	12–15 reps, holding 5lb (2kg) weights: 1–2 sets
LEVEL 3	8–12 reps, holding 8lb (4kg) weights: 2–3 sets

1 From a seated position on the ball, roll down into bridge position with head, neck, and shoulders supported. Holding a free weight in your right hand, bend your elbow to 90 degrees. Brace the elbow with your left hand.

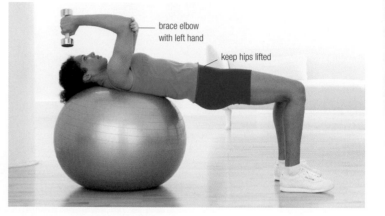

brace elbow with left hand

keep hips lifted

palm in, wrist straight

feel it here

2 Continuing to brace the back of your elbow with your left hand, exhale and straighten the arm to the ceiling. Repeat the movement as directed, switch arms and repeat.

head, neck, and shoulders supported

knees over ankles

Biceps curl

The biceps is one of the first muscles to respond with training and it makes life easier when you have to pull, lift, or carry a load. Resting your foot on an unstable surface such as the ball as you do the exercise will help improve your core stability and balance.

Begin at Level 1 and progress at your own pace to Levels 2 & 3	
LEVEL 1	10 reps, holding 3lb (1kg) weights: 1–2 sets
LEVEL 2	12–15 reps, holding 5lb (2kg) weights: 1–2 sets
LEVEL 3	8–12 reps, holding 8–10lb (4–5kg) weights: 2–3 sets

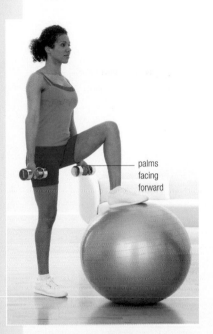

palms facing forward

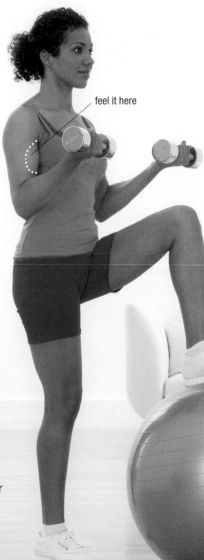

feel it here

feel it here

Easier alternative
If you find it hard to balance on one leg with the raised foot on the ball, practice the exercise standing on one leg on the floor.

1 Hold one free weight in each hand, arms by your sides and palms facing forward. Keeping the knee soft, balance on your right leg and rest your left foot on top of the ball.

2 Exhale and bend your elbows, bringing the weights up toward your shoulders. Pause, then inhale and slowly straighten your arms back to the starting position. Repeat the movement as directed.

Crunch and twist

Doing crunches on the ball is one of the best ways of targeting the abdominal muscles. Adding the twist recruits the obliques, while hugging the weight overloads the muscles to make them stronger, lending power to twisting and turning the torso, and keeping it erect.

Begin at Level 1 and progress at your own pace to Levels 2 & 3	
LEVEL 1	10 reps, holding one 3lb (1kg) weight: 1–2 sets
LEVEL 2	12–15 reps, holding one 5lb (2kg) weight: 1–2 sets
LEVEL 3	12–15 reps, holding one 8lb (4kg) weight: 1–2 sets

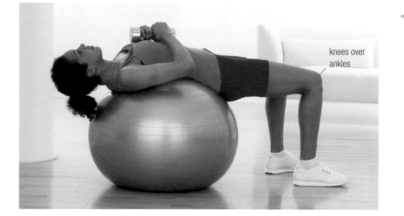

knees over ankles

1 From a seated position, roll down until your midback is supported on the ball. Keep your head and neck aligned with your spine and parallel to the floor. Hold one free weight in both hands, holding it vertically against your chest. Inhale.

keep elbows wide

2 As you exhale, contract the abs and lift your head and neck, twisting your left shoulder toward your right hip. Hold, then inhale and slowly release back to center. Repeat to the other side, then repeat as directed.

Push/pull on ball

This core strengthener engages the abdominals and spinal extensors (*see pp28–29*), and is an excellent alternative to endless crunches. If you have a spinal condition, it is a perfect way to train the abs without rounding the upper back, which can place stress on the vertebrae.

Begin at Level 1 and progress at your own pace to Levels 2 & 3	
LEVEL 1	10 reps: 1–2 sets
LEVEL 2	12–15 reps: 1–2 sets
LEVEL 3	20 reps: 1–2 sets

1 Kneeling in front of the ball with your knees hip-width apart, place your hands on top of the ball, close to you. Pull your abdominals tight and draw your shoulder blades down.

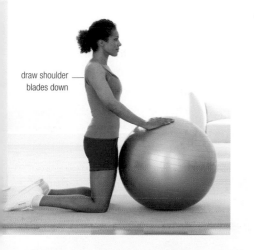

draw shoulder blades down

2 Push the ball away from you, dropping your hips as you shift your weight onto the ball. Then, using your abdominals, pull the ball back toward you, returning to an upright position. Repeat the movement as directed.

body in straight line from shoulder to knee

straight arms

feel it here

body at 45-degree angle to floor

Jackknife on ball

While this exercise works the entire abdominal area, you will feel it in your deepest abdominal muscle, the transversus abdominis (*see pp28–29*). Do not attempt the advanced version (*opposite*) until you are confident doing level 3 of this version.

Begin at Level 1 and progress at your own pace to Levels 2 & 3	
LEVEL 1	10 reps: 1–2 sets
LEVEL 2	12–15 reps: 1–2 sets
LEVEL 3	20 reps: 1–2 sets

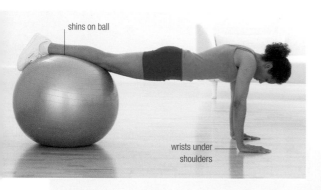

shins on ball

wrists under shoulders

1 Starting from a face-down position on the ball (*see pp34–35*), walk your hands forward until your wrists are directly under your shoulders and your shins are resting on top of the ball, legs and feet together. Your body should form a straight line from head to heels. Inhale.

pike hips

knees bent

2 As you exhale, tighten your abdominals and bend both knees in toward the chest, pulling the ball underneath you as you lift your hips. Inhale as you straighten your legs to roll the ball back to the start position. Repeat as directed, keeping head and spine aligned.

Easier alternative
If you're a beginner, use a modified range of motion: start with the ball under your thighs and roll it in from the knees instead of from the lower legs.

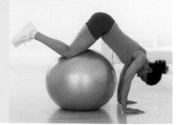

Advanced jackknife on ball

1 Walk out on the ball until your wrists are under your shoulders and your shins are on the ball. Use your abdominals to keep your lower back in line with your hips and shoulders. Inhale.

head, back, and legs aligned

JOAN'S TIP

Be sure to keep your head and neck aligned with your spine as you invert your torso.

2 Exhale as you pull your abs tight and pike your hips to the ceiling in one fluid movement so that your body forms an inverted "V," with the tops of your feet resting on the ball. Pause, then inhale and slowly return to the starting position to repeat.

pike hips

tops of feet on ball

THE **26-35** WARM-UP

This is an advanced warm-up that requires a base of leg strength and healthy knees. Different variations of the lunge combined with upper body movements create a full-body "pump" that will reflect in a strong heartbeat and increased rate of breathing. When you begin, it is easier to learn the lunge variations first, then add the upper body movements.

Lunge: modified range of motion

Lunge: full range of motion

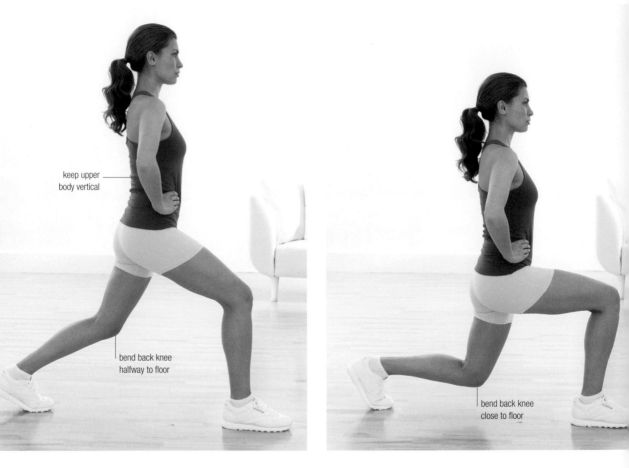

keep upper body vertical

bend back knee halfway to floor

bend back knee close to floor

If you are just beginning, or have knee problems, do the exercises in this warm-up with a modified range of motion, bending your knees just halfway to the floor. It you have any knee pain, skip these lunges and try a different warm-up, such as the step-touches (*pp38–43*) or step-ups (*pp58–64*).

If you are fit and healthy with no knee problems, and you are already strong in your legs, you can use a full range of motion when performing the lunges in this warm-up. Bend the back knee to within 3–4in (8–10cm) of the floor, always keeping your front knee bent at a right angle directly over the ankle.

Front lunge

raise arms
overhead

shift weight
to left leg

2 Inhale as you step forward with the right leg, bending both knees toward the floor; at the same time raise both arms overhead. Be careful to keep your front knee directly over your ankle. Exhale as you spring back to the starting position. Switch sides and repeat.
• **Reps** Do 10 reps of each position (one rep = both sides)

1 Stand with your feet parallel, hip-width apart, and with your arms relaxed by your sides. Shift your weight to your left, supporting leg.

right knee
over ankle

left knee down
toward floor

Diagonal lunge

1 Start from the center position, feet together, arms by your sides (*inset*). Pivot on your right foot; then, leading with the left leg, lunge out on a diagonal to 11 o'clock position. At the same time, lift your arms to the front and rotate your torso to face the direction of the lunge.

lunge out to 11 o' clock

torso rotated in direction of lunge

pivot on ball of foot

JOAN'S TIP

As you pivot your back foot in the direction of the lunge, keep proper alignment of foot-to-ankle-to-knee-to-hip

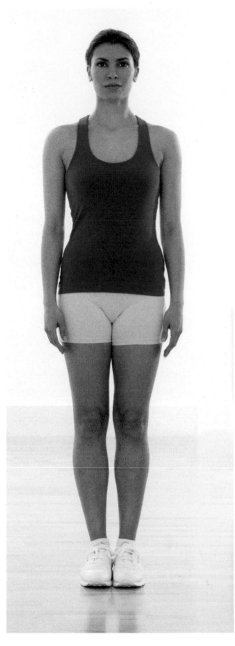

palms
facing in

lunge out to
1 o' clock

knee in line with
foot and ankle

2 Exhale as you spring back, pivoting your foot to return to the center position. With your feet together and arms by your sides, prepare to lunge to the other side.

3 Pivot on your left foot and lunge out with your right leg to 1 o'clock position, lifting your arms to shoulder height and rotating your torso in the direction of the lunge. Continue lunging to alternate sides as directed.
• **Reps** Do 10 reps of each position (one rep = both sides)

Side lunge

26-35

The working leg bends as you lunge to the side; the standing leg remains straight.

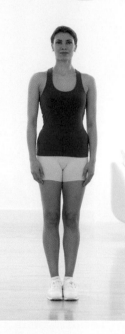

reach left arm overhead

Starting from the center position (*inset*), lunge to the left (9 o'clock), leading with the left leg and bending your knee directly over the ankle. At the same time, reach your left arm overhead toward the center. Keep your right, supporting leg, straight. Exhale and return to center; inhale as you lunge to the right (3 o'clock), leading with the right leg and reaching the right arm overhead.

• **Reps** Do 10 reps of each position (one rep = both sides)

left knee bent over ankle

right leg straight

Reverse lunge

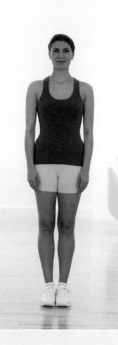

Starting in the center position (*inset*), step back with the right leg, bend both knees, simultaneously raising your arms overhead, palms in. Exhale and spring back to center, lowering your arms as you come forward. Switch sides and repeat as directed.

• **Reps** Do 10 reps of each position (one rep = both sides)

left knee bent over ankle

step back with right leg

THE **26-35** PROGRAM

Lifting free weights is like a sport, training your muscles as well as your balance and coordination. This challenging series of exercises requires core strength, especially to support the lower back in the bent-over positions. If you have any spinal condition, perform the seated modifications or choose one of the other resistance programs.

Mini-squat with overhead press

By combining upper and lower body moves with balance training, this full-body exercise recruits diverse muscle groups to function as a unit. Single arm and leg exercises are good core challengers because your trunk keeps you stable as you move your limbs.

Begin at Level 1 and progress at your own pace to Levels 2 & 3	
LEVEL 1	10 reps, holding 3lb (1kg) weights: 1–2 sets
LEVEL 2	12–15 reps, holding 5lb (2kg) weights: 1–2 sets
LEVEL 3	8–12 reps, holding 8lb (4kg) weights: 2–3 sets

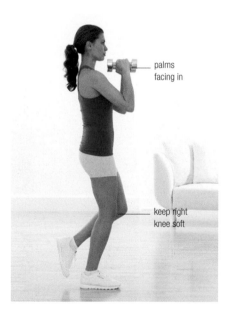

palms facing in

keep right knee soft

arms straight but not stiff

feel it here

1 Balance on the right leg. Tighten your abs and squeeze the glutes in your buttocks to stabilize your torso. Hold a weight in each hand in front of the shoulders, elbows close to your sides.

2 Inhale, maintaining your balance on your right leg. Then, as you exhale, slowly extend your arms to the ceiling. Pause for a moment.

3 As you inhale, lower the weights to shoulder level and, still balancing, bend your right leg into a mini-squat position. Exhale as you straighten the leg and repeat the sequence without touching the foot down. Repeat as directed, switch sides and repeat.

JOAN'S TIP

Reach back with your hips as you bend your knee to keep it in line with your toes.

keep foot off the floor

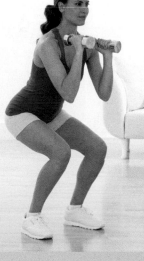

Easier alternative
If you find it difficult to perform this exercise while standing on one leg, begin by practicing the sequence with both feet flat on the floor until your legs become stronger.

Dead lift

The action here is to flex forward from the hip, keeping the spine straight, then return to an upright position. It's a good strengthening stimulus for the muscles of the spine, the gluteus maximus, and the hamstrings (see pp28–29). Do not try this if you have lower back problems.

Begin at Level 1 and progress at your own pace to Levels 2 & 3	
LEVEL 1	10 reps, holding 5lb (2kg) weights: 1–2 sets
LEVEL 2	12–15 reps, 8lb (4g) weights: 1–2 sets
LEVEL 3	8–12 reps, 10–12lb (5–5.5kg) weights: 2–3 sets

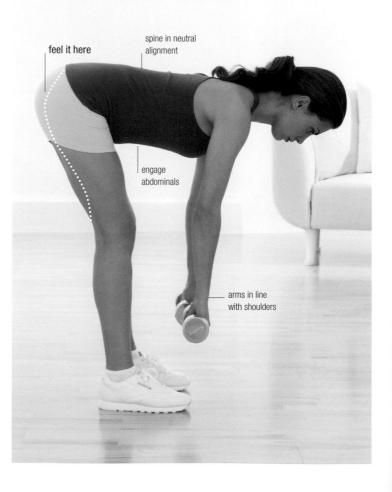

palms facing back

knees straight but not locked

feet parallel, hip-width apart

2 Bend forward from the hips, lowering the weights below your knees, close to your shins, until you feel your hamstrings stretch. Contract the glutes (see pp28–29), exhale, and straighten up to the starting position. Repeat the movement as directed.

feel it here

spine in neutral alignment

engage abdominals

arms in line with shoulders

1 Stand with your feet parallel, hip-width apart, knees straight, but not stiff. Hold a free weight in each hand in front of your thighs, arms straight, palms facing back. Engage your abdominals to maintain neutral spine alignment.

Back leg lift

This is a great exercise for developing strength and balance throughout the body. Your core muscles work to stabilize your torso as you lengthen into the lay-out position, the back leg lift targets the hamstrings and glutes, and holding the weights adds work to the upper body.

Begin at Level 1 and progress at your own pace to Levels 2 & 3	
LEVEL 1	10 reps, holding 5lb (2kg) weights: 1–2 sets
LEVEL 2	12–15 reps, holding 8lb (4kg) weights: 1–2 sets
LEVEL 3	20 reps, holding 10lb (5kg) weights: 1–2 sets

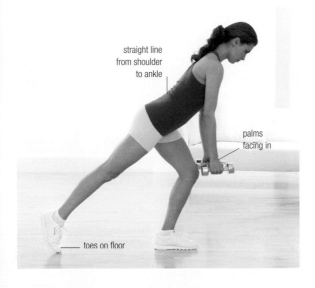

straight line from shoulder to ankle

palms facing in

toes on floor

1 Holding a free weight in each hand, stand with all your weight on your left leg, knee bent. Straighten your spine and bend forward from the hip as you extend the right leg behind you, resting the toes lightly on the floor to create a straight line from your shoulder to your foot.

feel it here

2 Continue to hinge forward from the hip until your back is nearly parallel to the floor. Keeping your hips square and right leg straight, lift your right leg to hip height. Lower the right foot to the floor without touching it, then lift again. Repeat all reps on one side, then switch sides and repeat.

Plié with front shoulder raise

The turn-out of the plié squat engages the adductors of the inner thighs, as well as glutes, hamstrings, and quads. For maximum benefit, squeeze the inner thighs and buttocks as you straighten your legs. Adding the front shoulder raise gives you two exercises in one.

Begin at Level 1 and progress at your own pace to Levels 2 & 3	
LEVEL 1	10 reps, holding one 5lb (2kg) weight: 1–2 sets
LEVEL 2	12–15 reps, holding one 8lb (4kg) weight: 1–2 sets
LEVEL 3	8–12 reps, holding one 10lb (5kg) weight: 2–3 sets

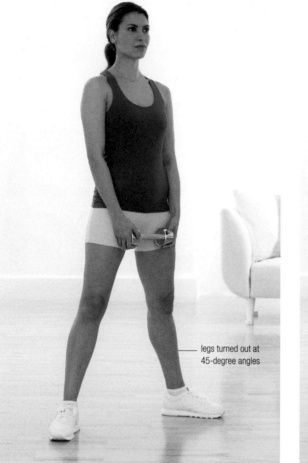

legs turned out at 45-degree angles

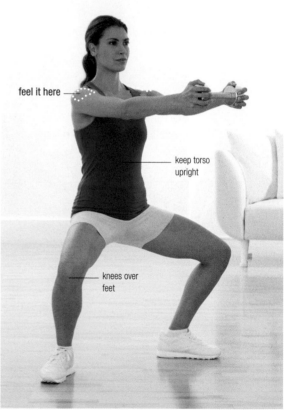

feel it here

keep torso upright

knees over feet

1 Stand with your feet slightly wider than hip-width apart. Shift your weight back to your heels and turn both legs out, with the feet at 45-degree angles. Hold one free weight as shown, with arms straight down to the front.

2 As you inhale bend your knees until the thighs are parallel to the floor; simultaneously lift the weight to chest height. Exhale and tighten the buttocks and inner thighs as you return to the starting position. Repeat as directed.

Bent-over alternating lat row

To sculpt a trim, tight torso you need to include exercises that train the lats (*see pp28-29*), the muscles that give the back a defined "V" shape. As they firm up you will get a smoother line in clothing and your whole body will take on a different appearance as your posture improves.

Begin at Level 1 and progress at your own pace to Levels 2 & 3	
LEVEL 1	10 reps, holding 5lb (2kg) weights: 1–2 sets
LEVEL 2	12–15 reps, holding 8lb (4kg) weights: 1–2 sets
LEVEL 3	8–12 reps, 10–12lb (5–5.5kg) weights: 2–3 sets

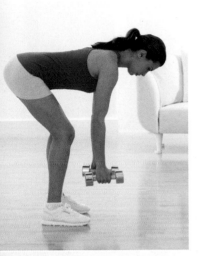

1 Bend forward from the hips until your back is parallel to the floor. Be sure to keep your back straight while maintaining the slight curve in the lower back. Hold one free weight in each hand, arms extended toward the floor, palms facing in.

feel it here

keep bent elbow close to the side

feel it here

2 Pull your right shoulder blade in toward the spine to anchor it, then bend your right elbow and draw the free weight up toward your waist, keeping the elbow in close to your side. Slowly straighten your right arm toward the floor and repeat with the left arm. (This makes one rep). Repeat as directed, alternating sides.

Beginner's alternative
If you don't have the core strength to perform the exercise as shown, you will still get all the benefits by doing it sitting in a chair.

Reverse fly/shoulder extension

Daily habits of slouching over desks, computers, steering wheels, or baby carriages have a cumulative effect on our posture. This combination move targets key postural muscles as well as the difficult areas of the back of the upper arm.

Begin at Level 1 and progress at your own pace to Levels 2 & 3	
LEVEL 1	10 reps, holding 3lb (1kg) weights: 1 set
LEVEL 2	12–15 reps, holding 5lb (2kg) weights: 1 set
LEVEL 3	8–12 reps, holding 8lb (4kg) weights: 1 set

1 Holding a light free weight in each hand with your palms facing in, straighten your spine then flex forward from the hips in neutral spine alignment until your torso is nearly parallel to the floor.

2 Inhale, then, as you exhale, raise your arms out to the sides in line with your shoulders and to shoulder height. Keep your elbows slightly rounded and your wrists straight. Maintain the spine in neutral alignment, and the knees slightly bent.

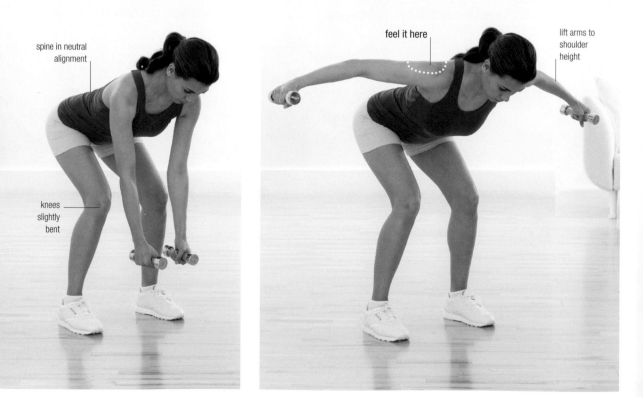

spine in neutral alignment

knees slightly bent

feel it here

lift arms to shoulder height

3 Inhale and slowly lower the weights to the starting position with the arms straight and the palms facing in. Check that the spine is still in neutral alignment.

arms straight

palms facing in

lift arms above back

feel it here

4 On the next exhalation, lift your arms behind you, coming up slightly above the level of your back. The arms are straight but not stiff and the spine is in neutral alignment. Repeat the sequence as directed.

knees slightly bent

JOAN'S TIP

If you find the combination too taxing, perform each exercise separately.

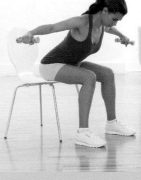

Easier alternative
If you have any back problems or do not have the core strength to stabilize your torso in the standing position, perform this exercise while seated in a chair.

Push-up with a touch

Begin this advanced push-up kneeling on the floor, your hands 3–4in (8–10cm) wider and slightly in front of your shoulders. Use your abs to keep your back straight. You can rest your lower legs on the floor or bend them and cross the ankles (as I prefer).

Begin at Level 1 and progress at your own pace to Levels 2 & 3	
LEVEL 1	5–8 reps (1 rep = both sides): 1 set
LEVEL 2	10–12 reps: 1 set
LEVEL 3	15–20 reps: 1 set

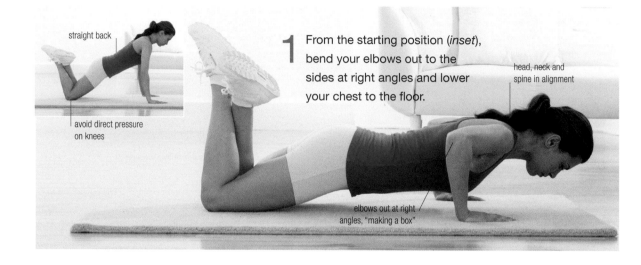

straight back

avoid direct pressure on knees

1 From the starting position (*inset*), bend your elbows out to the sides at right angles and lower your chest to the floor.

head, neck and spine in alignment

elbows out at right angles, "making a box"

2 Exhale and straighten your arms to press up to the starting position. At the top, cross your right hand over to tap the left hand then return to the starting position. Repeat as directed, alternating sides.

tap left hand with right

Kneeling triceps kickback

The classic kickback exercise isolates the triceps in one simple move of the arm. This version makes it more interesting by involving the whole body. As your muscles work in concert to balance and stabilize, they function more closely to the way they do in daily life.

Begin at Level 1 and progress at your own pace to Levels 2 & 3	
LEVEL 1	10 reps, holding 3lb (1kg) weight: 1–2 sets
LEVEL 2	12–15 reps, holding 5lb (2kg) weight: 1–2 sets
LEVEL 3	8–12 reps, holding 8–10lb (4–5kg) weight: 1–2 sets

1 Kneeling on all fours, extend the left leg to the back at hip height. Holding a free weight in the right hand, bend your elbow to 90 degrees, anchoring your upper arm close to your side, parallel to the floor.

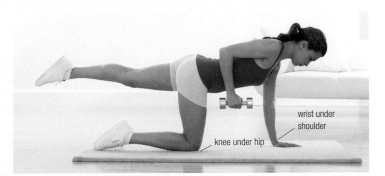

wrist under shoulder

knee under hip

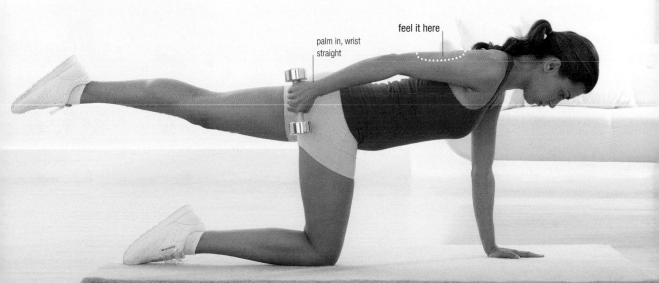

feel it here

palm in, wrist straight

2 Exhale and straighten your right arm to the back, without locking the elbow, then return to the starting position with the elbow bent at 90 degrees. Repeat as directed, switch sides and repeat.

JOAN'S TIP

Ensure that your shoulders and hips are square to the floor and your torso parallel to the floor.

Concentration curl

Working one arm at a time in a concentrated fashion will highlight any imbalances in strength between the two sides of your body. To even things out, start with your weaker side, work the dominant side next, then return and do an extra set on your weaker side.

Begin at Level 1 and progress at your own pace to Levels 2 & 3	
LEVEL 1	10 reps, holding 5lb (2kg) weight: 1–2 sets
LEVEL 2	12–15 reps, holding 8lb (4kg) weight: 1–2 sets
LEVEL 3	8–12 reps, holding 10lb (5kg) weight: 2–3 sets

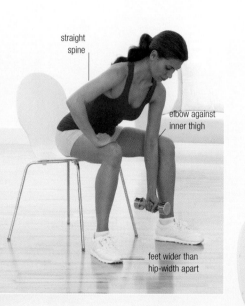

straight spine

elbow against inner thigh

feet wider than hip-width apart

1 Holding a free weight in your left hand, sit forward on a chair. Place your right hand on top of your right thigh and lean forward from the hip. Brace the back of your left elbow against your left inner thigh and extend your left arm toward the floor, palm facing in. Inhale.

2 As you exhale, bend your left elbow and contract the biceps to bring the weight up toward your shoulder. Pause, then slowly lower the weight to the starting position, maintaining tension in the muscle. Repeat as directed then switch sides and repeat.

feel it here

flat wrist

Full crunch

This is an efficient variation of the crunch because it combines working the upper and the lower portions of the rectus abdominis (see pp28–29) in one move. Once you start working, keep tension in the muscle by never relaxing back to the starting position.

Begin at Level 1 and progress at your own pace to Levels 2 & 3	
LEVEL 1	10 reps: 1–2 sets
LEVEL 2	12–15 reps: 1–2 sets
LEVEL 3	20 reps: 1–2 sets

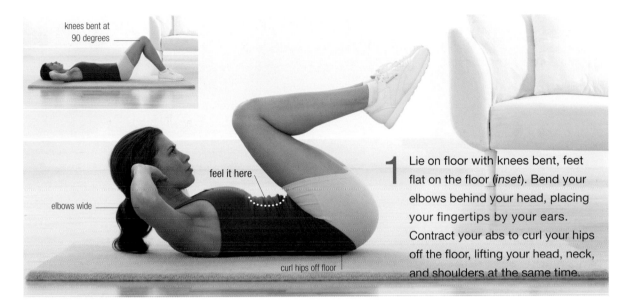

knees bent at 90 degrees

feel it here

elbows wide

curl hips off floor

1 Lie on floor with knees bent, feet flat on the floor (inset). Bend your elbows behind your head, placing your fingertips by your ears. Contract your abs to curl your hips off the floor, lifting your head, neck, and shoulders at the same time.

2 Keep your head lifted as you release your shoulders and hips back to the floor, lightly tapping down with your toes. Repeat the movement as directed.

head stays lifted

keep abs contracted

Torso twist with weight

The twisting motion of this exercise targets the obliques (*see pp28–29*) that run along the sides of the waist, firming them and giving a sleeker line to your torso. Initiate the upper and lower body rotations with your core by pulling your belly button in toward your spine.

Begin at Level 1 and progress at your own pace to Levels 2 & 3	
LEVEL 1	10 reps, holding 3lb (1kg) weight: 1–2 sets
LEVEL 2	12–15 reps, holding 5lb (2kg) weight: 1–2 sets
LEVEL 3	12–15 reps, holding 8lb (4kg) weight: 1–2 sets

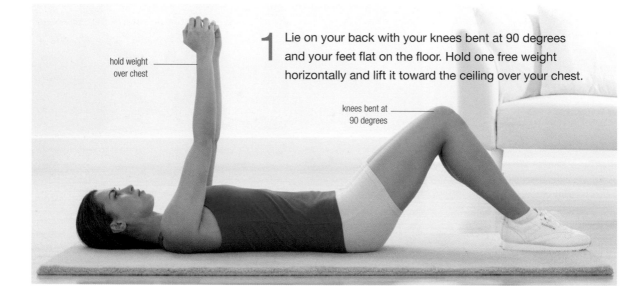

hold weight over chest

knees bent at 90 degrees

1 Lie on your back with your knees bent at 90 degrees and your feet flat on the floor. Hold one free weight horizontally and lift it toward the ceiling over your chest.

2 Rotate your upper body to the right, reaching across chest with left arm and bending right arm to lower the weight toward the floor. At the same time, drop both knees to the left. Repeat to the other side (this makes one rep). Repeat, alternating sides.

twist upper body to right

feel it here

drop knees to left

Torso twist with weight: advanced

This variation increases the resistance by raising the legs and curling the upper body off the floor. Squeeze thighs and lower legs together, stabilize the torso, then use your breathing to establish the rhythm, moving your arms and legs in a coordinated, rhythmic fashion.

Begin at Level 1 and progress at your own pace to Levels 2 & 3	
LEVEL 1	10 reps, holding 3lb (1kg) weight: 1–2 sets
LEVEL 2	12–15 reps, holding 5lb (2kg) weight: 1–2 sets
LEVEL 3	12–15 reps, holding 8lb (4kg) weight: 1–2 sets

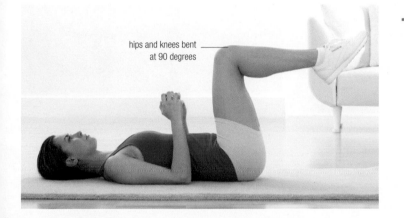

hips and knees bent at 90 degrees

1 Lie on your back with your knees bent over your hips, feet in the air, lower legs parallel to the floor. Hold one free weight horizontally over your chest with your elbows bent at 90 degrees. Inhale, then as you exhale, compress your abdomen to stabilize your back on the floor. Inhale again.

2 As you exhale, curl your upper body forward, straightening the arms and reaching the weight to the outside of the right thigh. At the same time rotate your legs to the left, keeping your knees and ankles together. Inhale as you return to center then exhale as you switch sides to repeat. (This makes one rep). Repeat as directed.

keep feet and ankles together

reach arms to the right

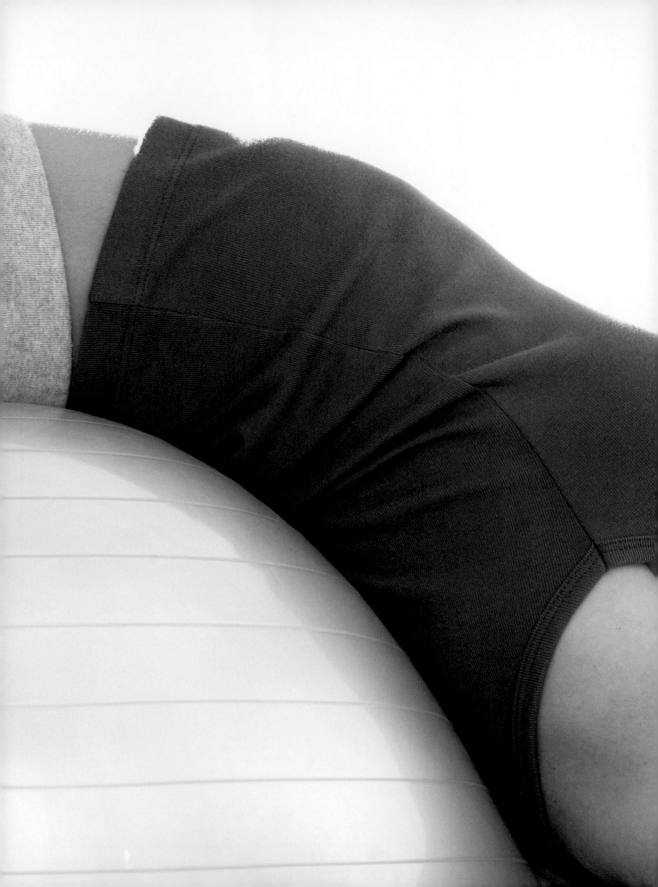

Stretching energizes the body and defends against aging by lengthening the muscles to keep you tall and straight. Being flexible makes you agile, keeping your movements fluid and youthful.

flexibility
training

INTRODUCING **FLEXIBILITY**

Decreased flexibility may be a common aspect of aging—but it is one that you can do something about, no matter what your age. Just a few minutes of daily stretching can help maintain flexibility, which in turn keeps the muscles supple and counteracts the wear and tear of everyday life, allowing you to maintain a youthful appearance and active lifestyle.

What is flexibility?

Your ability to stretch depends on genetics as well as your daily habits. The unique structure of bones and the length of the soft tissue (muscles, tendons, and ligaments) surrounding them determine the joints' range of movement. Some joints, like those affected by arthritis, may be "stiff" or restricted; others, like those of a contortionist, "loose" or hypermobile. Each one of us, however, must have enough flexibility to function effectively in our day-to-day activities.

The benefits of stretching

Nothing ages our demeanor more than poor posture and short, jerky movements. The constant downward pull of gravity and gradual dehydration of the body's tissues cause us literally to shrink over time, but stretching can help restore lost height by lengthening the muscles around the spine and improving the mobility of the upper back. No beauty product will take years of your age as efficiently as just standing up a little straighter.

Muscles maintain the alignment of the skeleton in all positions. There is a natural tendency for some muscles to be short and tight, with others prone to being long and weak. Stretching can help offset this imbalance and improve the alignment, as in the "forward slouch." We see this all the time: a stooped posture with the upper back rounded, shoulders hunched, and the head forward of the body. The remedy is to stretch the chest and shoulder muscles (which are short and tight) and strengthen the neck and back muscles (which are long and weak).

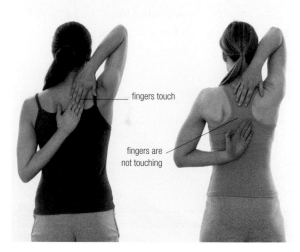

fingers touch

fingers are not touching

The ability to stretch *is individual, some of us being naturally more flexible than others. You may also find that you are more flexible on one side than the other. Try this stretch for yourself.*

Preventing pain, injury, and stress

Poor posture and alignment can cause pain when the muscles become chronically tired and strained and more prone to injury. Headache, neck and shoulder tension, sciatica, and hip and knee pain can all be symptoms of this. In addition, shortened muscles are more at risk for injury caused by simple movements. By enhancing our mobility, however, stretching increases our efficiency in all activities so that they require less effort and leave us feeling less tired.

Stretching also energizes us by releasing tension from the muscles and refreshing the mind. As anyone who has practiced yoga knows, holding a stretch position is a type of moving meditation that reduces stress and promotes relaxation.

How to stretch

I am a strong advocate of static stretching, where the idea is to coax the muscle into lengthening. Slowly stretch until you feel "gentle pulling" in the belly of the muscle, without any pain. Hold this position: when the muscle is first stretched, nerve impulses signal the muscle to contract to prevent overstretching, but after about 20 seconds, the nerve impulses diminish and the muscle relaxes, allowing you to go a little deeper into the stretch. To avoid injury, move gradually and never twist, turn, or bounce while in a stretch.

Cold muscles are less pliable and resist stretching, so warm up first with five minutes of light jogging or rhythmic limbering exercises. Always stretch after exercising to put length into the muscles you have worked and to prevent tight, sore muscles.

Focus on the muscle you are targeting and pay attention to stabilizing the rest of the body. Take your time and remember to breathe. Some people find stretching stressful (usually they have tight muscles) and breathing helps you relax into the stretch as well as advance deeper into the position.

flexible lower back

less flexible lower back

hand touches the floor

hand doesn't reach floor

Genetics and lifestyle influence your level of flexibility. Even if you are not naturally flexible, you can improve and benefit with regular stretching. Make it a daily habit.

THE 56–65 **STRETCHES**

Practice these exercises regularly to increase the flexibility in your lower back and hamstrings (*see pp28–29*), and to improve your score on the Sit-and-reach test (*see pp22–23*). The Pelvic tilt combines abdominal compression with a slight rotation of the hips, both strengthening the abdomen and stretching the lumbar spine.

Pelvic tilt

1 Lie on your back with your knees bent, feet on the floor, and arms by your sides. Your spine should be in neutral alignment with a slight natural curve in the lower back. Inhale and bring the breath into your abdomen, filling the belly with air.

abdomen inflated

spine in neutral alignment

2 Exhale forcefully, pulling the abs in tight. In one fluid motion, flatten your lower back to the floor and curl your hips 1in (2.5cm) off the floor. Hold for 3 seconds, slowly release back to starting position, then repeat.
• **Reps** Do 15–20 reps

pull abs tight

feel it here

curl hips off floor

Knee to shoulder

Start as for Pelvic tilt (*opposite*). Inhale as you clasp your hands around the thigh; as you exhale, pull the knee toward your shoulder. Hold for 10 seconds. Return to starting position, switch sides, and repeat.
• **Reps** Do 1–3 reps (1 rep = both sides)

feel it here

Double knee to chest

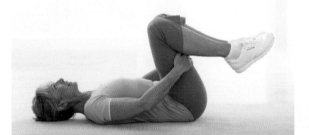

1 Starting as above, bring your right thigh up over your chest, holding underneath with your right hand; then, with your left hand, pull your left knee up in line with the right knee. Separate the knees slightly.

2 Inhale then, as you exhale, pull both knees toward your shoulders, curling the tailbone 1in (2.5cm) off the mat. Hold for 3 seconds then release your hips to the floor and repeat.
• **Reps** Do 1–3 reps

feel it here

curl hips off floor

feel it here

Hamstring stretch

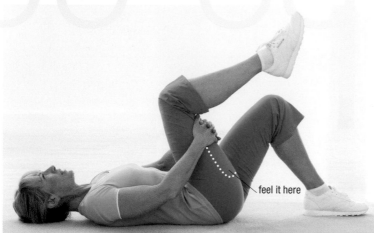

feel it here

1 Lie on your back with knees bent at 90 degrees, feet flat on the floor. Maintaining the right angle at your knee, clasp your hands underneath your right thigh and gently pull the knee toward the chest. If your hamstrings are tight, you will begin to feel the stretch in this position; otherwise, continue to the full stretch in step 2.

Increased stretch
Extend the left leg as you raise the right leg to the ceiling—but only do this if you can keep the right knee straight and maintain the 90-degree angle.

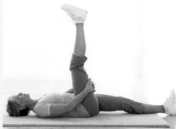

2 Straighten your right knee so that the right thigh is at 90 degrees (or more) to the floor. Hold for 20–30 seconds, then lower your foot to the floor, switch sides, and repeat.

• **Reps** Do 1–3 reps (1 rep = both sides)

feel it here

relax neck and shoulders

Knee drop

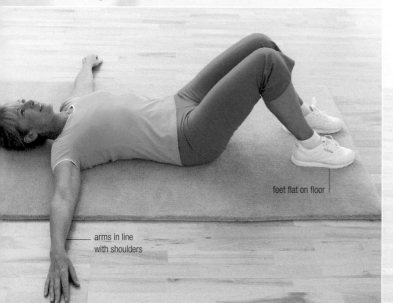

feet flat on floor

arms in line
with shoulders

1 Lie on your back with both knees
bent at 90 degrees. Feet are flat
on the floor, arms outstretched in
line with your shoulders, and
palms down.

turn head to left

keep feet
together

drop knees to right

2 Keeping knees and feet together, drop both
knees to the floor to the right and turn your
head in the opposite direction. Hold the
position for 20–30 seconds then change
sides and repeat.

• **Reps** Do 1–3 reps (1 rep = both sides)

Sphinx

1 Lie face down on a mat with a folded towel under your forehead to ensure proper alignment of your head and neck with your spine. Bend your arms and rest your forearms on the floor, palms down. Pull your belly button toward your spine.

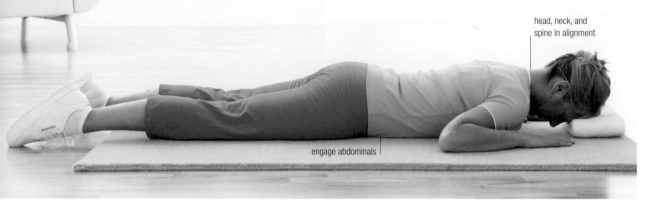

head, neck, and spine in alignment

engage abdominals

2 Lengthen the spine by reaching forward with the top of the head. Draw your shoulder blades down and together. Slide your elbows forward so that they are directly under your shoulders as you lift your torso. Keep your hips pressed into the floor. Breathe naturally throughout. Hold the position for 20–30 seconds.

feel it here

feel it here

hips pressed into floor

elbows under shoulders

Child's pose

1 Kneel on a mat or a well-padded surface, with your knees under your hips and your wrists under your shoulders. Keep your nose down to ensure that your head and neck are aligned with your spine.

head and neck aligned with spine

2 Sit back on your heels and bend forward until your forehead is resting on the mat, your arms reaching forward. Allow your body to relax and sink down into the position. Hold the position for 20–30 seconds.

feel it here

forehead resting on mat

Arch and curve

1 Kneel on the floor with your knees under your hips and your wrists under your shoulders. Keep your nose down to maintain proper alignment of your head, neck, and spine. Your back should be straight, with a slight natural curve in the lumbar spine.

nose down

wrists under shoulders

knees under hips

2 Breathing naturally throughout, round your back up toward the ceiling, letting your head drop forward and tucking your hips under to create an arch.

feel it here

tuck hips under

let head drop forward

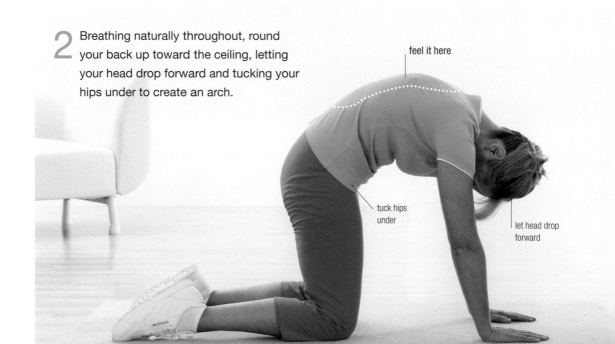

3 Reverse the position by bringing your head up and curving your low back into a "C" shape. If you have any lower back problems, just bring the spine into neutral flat back position without hyperextending it.

• **Reps** Do 1–3 reps

bring head up

curve back into "C" shape

feel it here

JOAN'S TIP

If you have a lower back problem, stay within a pain-free range of motion while exercising.

THE **46-55** STRETCHES

Make stretching a daily habit to stay limber as you age, especially if you tend to be stiff. Because the muscle groups of the legs are larger than those of the upper body, the leg stretches (*pp132–133*) should be held for 20–30 seconds, allowing time for the muscle to lengthen. Breathe into the stretch, using the exhale to move deeper into the position.

Chest stretch

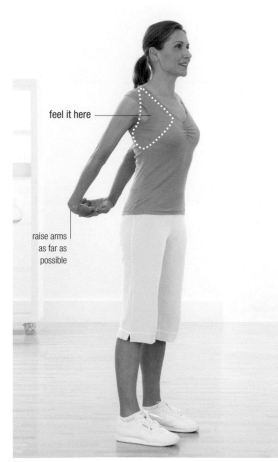

feel it here

raise arms as far as possible

Midback/rear shoulder stretch

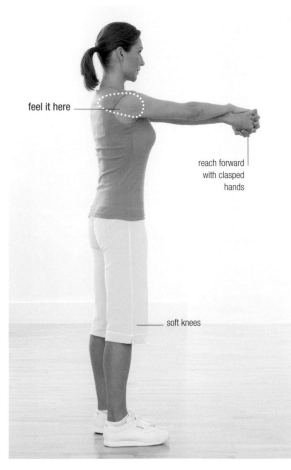

feel it here

reach forward with clasped hands

soft knees

Stand up tall, lengthening through the spine. Lift your chest and relax your shoulders. Look straight ahead, keeping your chin level. Clasp your hands behind your back and slowly raise your arms as far as possible. Hold for 10-15 seconds, breathing naturally.
• **Reps** Do 1–2 reps

With your spine straight, extend your arms to the front at shoulder level. Crisscross your wrists and clasp your hands together, thumbs pointing to the floor. Slide your shoulder blades apart and reach as far forward as possible. Hold for 10–15 seconds.
• **Reps** Do 1–2 reps

Lat stretch

Triceps stretch into side bend

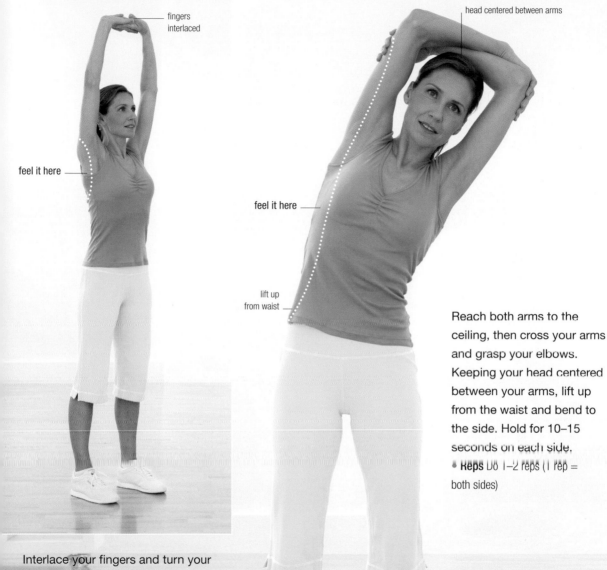

fingers interlaced

feel it here

head centered between arms

feel it here

lift up from waist

Reach both arms to the ceiling, then cross your arms and grasp your elbows. Keeping your head centered between your arms, lift up from the waist and bend to the side. Hold for 10–15 seconds on each side.
- **Reps** Do 1–2 reps (1 rep = both sides)

Interlace your fingers and turn your palms away from you. Straighten your elbows then raise your arms to the ceiling, reaching as high as you can. Hold for 10-15 seconds.
- **Reps** Do 1–2 reps

Calf stretch

use wall for support

feel it here

lower heel off edge of step

Stand on the edge of the step. Wrap the toes of your right foot around the back of your left ankle then lower your left heel toward the floor. Hold the stretch for 20–30 seconds without bouncing. Repeat on the other side.

• **Reps** Do 1–2 reps (1 rep = both sides)

Quad stretch

Stand with your feet parallel, hip-width apart. Bend your right leg up toward your buttocks and hold the foot (or ankle, if you can't reach the foot) with your right hand. Keep the knees aligned in front, with the supporting leg soft. Hold the stretch for 20–30 seconds without bouncing. Repeat on the other side.

• **Reps** Do 1–2 reps (1 rep = both sides)

hold foot or ankle

feel it here

keep knees aligned

Hip flexor stretch

Hamstring stretch

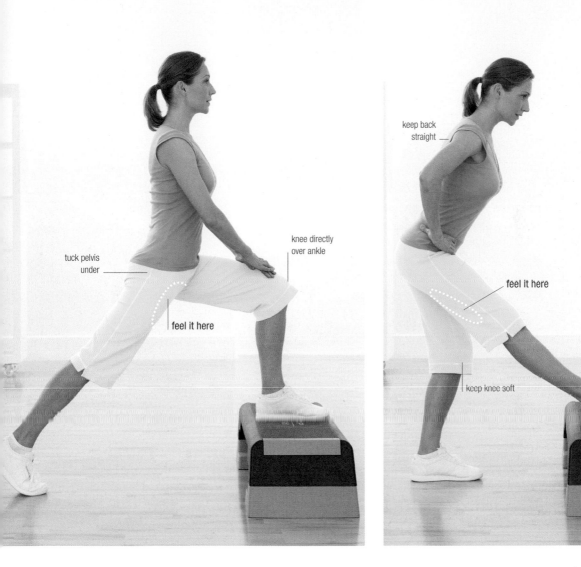

tuck pelvis under

knee directly over ankle

feel it here

keep back straight

feel it here

keep knee soft

Stand in a staggered lunge position with your left foot planted fully on the platform. Bend your left knee directly over the ankle and rest your hands on your thigh. Come up on the toes of the right foot and tuck your pelvis under to produce a stretch in the right hip flexor. Hold for 20–30 seconds without bouncing. Repeat on the other side.

• **Reps** Do 1–2 reps (1 rep = both sides)

Extend the right leg, resting the heel on the step with the toe pointing up. Soften the knee of the left leg. Stand up tall then flex forward from the hip, keeping your back straight. Hold for 20–30 seconds without bouncing. Repeat on other side.

• **Reps** Do 1–2 reps (1 rep = both sides)

THE **36–45** STRETCHES

Stretching on the ball can be very effective as the ball supports your body, relieving stress on the joints and allowing you to relax deeper into the positions. Make sure that you are securely positioned on the ball and that you use proper form to return to the starting position (*see pp34–35*). Remember to stretch both sides equally where applicable.

Full back bend over ball

Before you try this full spinal stretch, begin with the more conservative Supine chest stretch (*see inset*). If this is comfortable and you want a deeper stretch, reach your arms overhead and straighten your legs, rolling the ball down your spine as you arch over it. Extend your arms to the floor as far as is comfortable. Hold for 15–30 seconds.

• **Reps** Do one stretch

JOAN'S TIP

Caution: do not attempt this position if you have any problems with your back.

feet hip-width apart

fingertips to floor

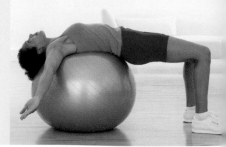

Supine chest stretch
Lie on the ball with head, neck, and shoulders fully supported and your hips lifted in a bridge. Stretch your arms out in a wide "V" above shoulder level, palms up. Shift the position of your arms to feel the stretch from various angles.

Child's pose into trunk rotation

1 Kneel on a padded surface with your knees hip-width apart and your arms outstretched on top of the ball, shoulder-width apart. Sit back on your heels and keep reaching forward until you feel a good stretch through your chest and shoulders. Hold the position for 15–30 seconds.

feel it here

knees hip-width apart

2 From the previous position, roll the ball to the right, rotating your trunk slightly. Your left hand will now be on top and your right hand near the floor. Keep your hips down, your weight back on your heels, and your head centered between your arms. Hold the position for 15–30 seconds, then switch sides.

• **Reps** Do one stretch in each position

head centered between arms

keep weight on heels

Seated oblique stretch

Seated hamstring stretch

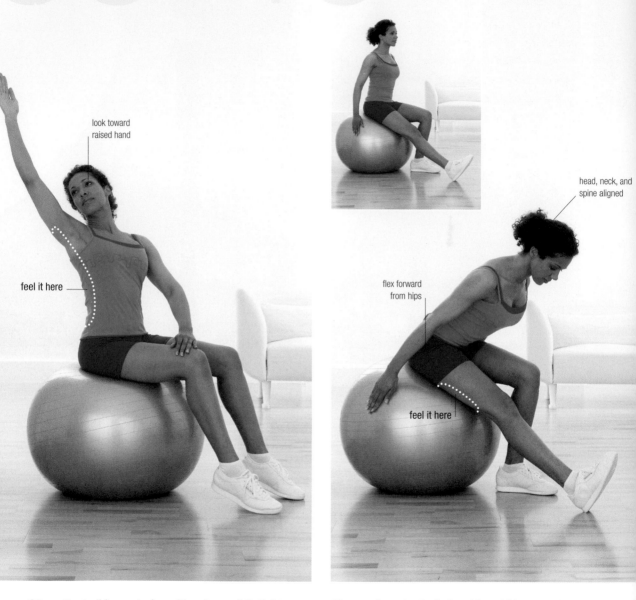

look toward
raised hand

feel it here

head, neck, and
spine aligned

flex forward
from hips

feel it here

Sit on the ball in neutral position (*see p34*); tighten your abs and lean back, keeping your spine straight. Lift up on your toes, reach your right arm overhead, and look up toward your raised hand. Cross your left arm to the right knee and turn into the stretch slightly. Hold for 15–30 seconds, then change sides.

• **Reps** Do one stretch on each side

Sit up tall on the ball, feet hip-width apart. Stretch your right leg out in front of you, keeping the left leg bent (*inset*). Lean forward from the hip, keeping your spine straight, until you feel pulling in the hamstring in the back of your right thigh. Hold for 15–30 seconds then repeat on the left.

• **Reps** Do one stretch on each side

Seated front hip stretch

Beginning in a sitting position, straighten your right leg behind you. Stabilize by pressing your toes into the floor. Keep your left leg bent to the front, knee over the ankle. To increase the stretch, roll the ball forward and hold for 15–30 seconds. Switch sides and repeat.

• **Reps** Do one stretch on each side

look straight ahead

feel it here

press toes into floor

JOAN'S TIP

Tucking your hips under will move the ball forward 1–2in (2.5–5cm) and increase the stretch.

Figure 4 (outer thigh) stretch

Begin in the supine position with your heels resting on top of the ball. Cross your left ankle over the right knee and pull the ball toward you with your right foot until you feel the stretch in your outer thigh. Hold for 15–30 seconds, then switch sides and repeat.

• **Reps** Do one stretch on each side

stretching left outer thigh

THE **26–35** STRETCHES

Based on yoga positions, this fluid sequence provides a full-body stretch as you progress through the movements. Instead of stretching body parts separately, the positions target multiple muscle groups, training your muscles to work in patterns and building flexibility and muscular balance simultaneously. Hold each position for 15–30 seconds.

Modified warrior sequence

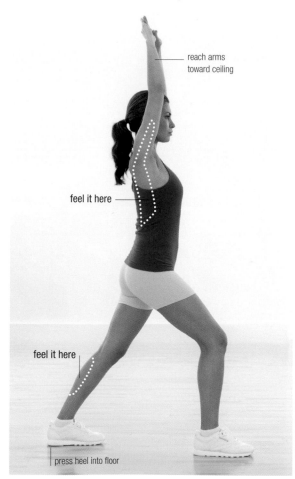

reach arms toward ceiling

feel it here

feel it here

press heel into floor

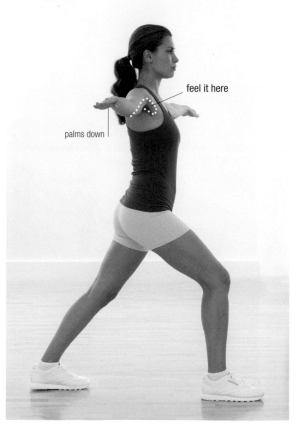

feel it here

palms down

1 Stand in a staggered lunge position, with the right leg forward. Straighten your back leg and press the heel into the floor. Interlock your thumbs and reach both arms to the ceiling. Keep your head centered between your elbows.

2 With your feet still in the staggered lunge position, right leg forward and left heel pressed into the floor, lower your arms out to the sides at shoulder level, palms down.

3 With your arms still out to the sides and your right foot pointing straight ahead, pivot your left foot outward to 90 degrees and turn your whole torso a quarter-turn to the left.

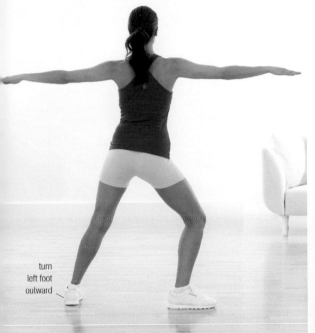

turn
left foot
outward

reach overhead
in side stretch

feel it here

4 Keeping your front knee bent, place your right hand on your right thigh for support and reach your left hand overhead in a side stretch.

Continued overleaf ▶

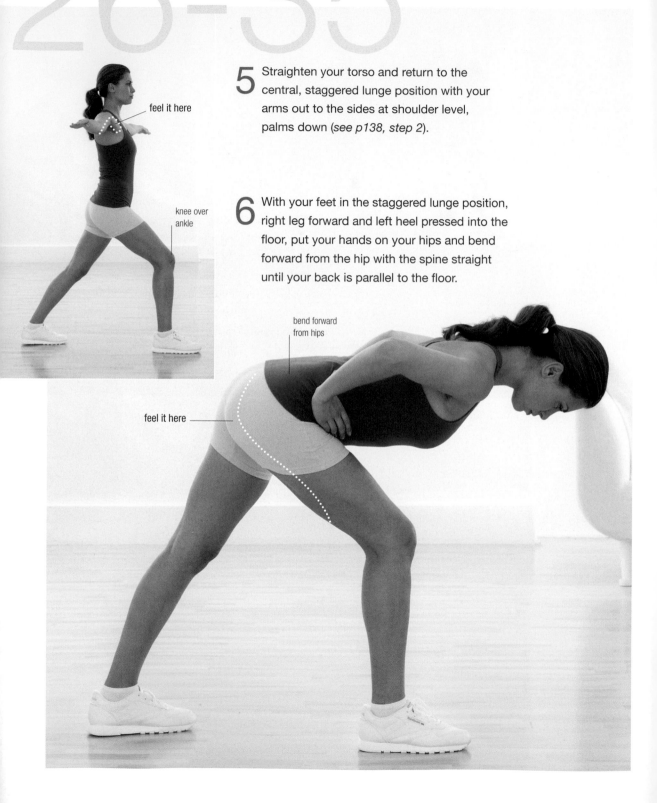

feel it here

knee over
ankle

5 Straighten your torso and return to the
central, staggered lunge position with your
arms out to the sides at shoulder level,
palms down (*see p138, step 2*).

6 With your feet in the staggered lunge position,
right leg forward and left heel pressed into the
floor, put your hands on your hips and bend
forward from the hip with the spine straight
until your back is parallel to the floor.

bend forward
from hips

feel it here

7 Return to an upright position and shift your weight forward onto the right leg. Balancing on the right leg, bend the left leg in a quad stretch; hold your left foot behind you with the left hand. Reach your right arm forward at shoulder level, palm down, for balance. Repeat whole sequence to the other side.

- **Reps** Do one sequence on each side, holding each position for 15–30 seconds

keep knees aligned

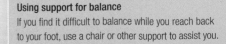

Using support for balance
If you find it difficult to balance while you reach back to your foot, use a chair or other support to assist you.

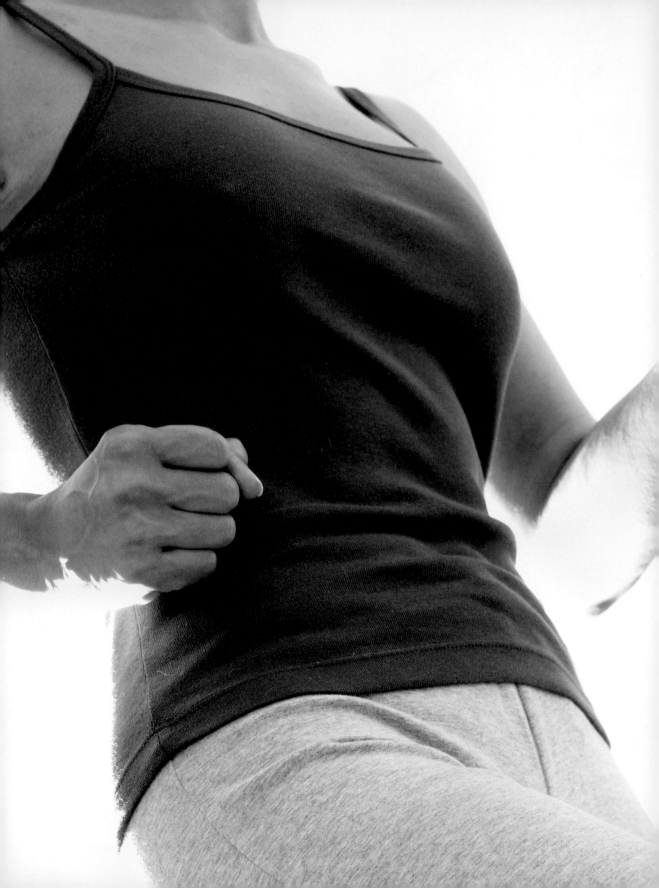

Your vitality and capacity for life depend on the efficiency of your cardiovascular system. The heart is a muscle that gets stronger with training, improving your ability to function day-to-day. The more you can do, the "younger" you are.

cardio training

INTRODUCING **CARDIO**

Cardiovascular fitness is one of the most important aspects of physical fitness. By strengthening your heart and lungs, regular cardio (or aerobic) exercise can increase your stamina, reduce your risk of heart disease, lower blood pressure, and improve cholesterol levels. A key factor in weight control, it will also help you firm up as you slim down.

A healthy heart is efficient, pumping more blood with each beat as it delivers oxygen to the working muscles. To become stronger, it must be exercised like any other muscle of the body, following the FIT guidelines of frequency, intensity and time (*see p12*).

Types of cardio (aerobic) exercise

Any activity that involves the continuous rhythmic contraction of large muscle groups (the legs, the back, the arms) for more than five minutes is considered aerobic, literally meaning "with oxygen."

This includes a wide range of activities such as dancing, brisk walking or hiking, jogging or running, cycling, skating, skiing, stair-climbing, and swimming, to name just a few.

I have chosen to use walking for our cardio programs, because it is a popular and universally available form of exercise. However, you can follow the same guidelines given in these programs for any aerobic activity of your choice. Each eight-week walking program has a different objective in terms of the cardio benefits you will achieve.

Heart rate target training zones (Karvonen method: 60–80 percent heart rate reserve)									
Resting heart rate	Age 25–29	30–34	35–39	40–44	45–49	50–54	55–59	60–64	over 65
under 50	133–164	130–160	127–156	124–152	121–148	118–144	115–140	112–136	109–134
50–54	135–165	132–161	129–157	126–153	123–149	120–145	117–141	114–137	111–135
55–59	137–166	134–162	131–158	128–154	125–150	122–146	119–142	116–138	113–136
60–64	139–167	136–163	133–159	130–155	127–151	124–147	121–143	118–139	115–137
65–69	141–168	138–164	135–160	132–156	129–152	126–148	123–144	120–140	117–138
70–74	143–169	140–165	137–161	134–157	131–153	128–149	125–145	122–141	119–139
75–79	145–170	142–166	139–162	136–158	133–154	130–150	127–146	124–142	121–140
80–85	147–171	144–167	141–163	138–159	135–155	132–151	129–147	126–143	123–141
over 85	149–172	146–168	143–164	140–160	137–156	134–152	131–148	128–144	125–142

How often, how hard, how long?

This depends on your goal. For health benefits, such as reducing your risk of heart disease, our national guidelines recommend a minimum of 30 minutes of brisk walking (or other light-to-moderate exercise) most days of the week. If you can't do it all at once, accumulate 30 minutes by doing it in shorter doses. Some experts recommend taking 10,000 steps (about 5 miles) each day. For cardiovascular conditioning, you need to do 20–30 minutes in your training range (*see chart opposite*) 3 times a week. For weight loss, 45–60 minutes of moderate intensity exercise every day are needed.

Establishing your training range

Your heart rate training range determines how hard you should work for light, moderate, and high intensity levels. The traditional, easy-to-use formula of "220 minus your age" gives an estimate of your maximum heart rate (EMHR)—that is, how fast your heart will beat during all-out exertion. Since nobody can sustain this level of exercise for long, we take 65–95 percent of EMHR to develop a training range with a continuum of low to high intensity.

For example, a 40-year-old woman has an EMHR of 180 beats per minute (220 minus 40). Her training range percentages are:

- 65 percent of 180 = 117
- 75 percent of 180 = 135
- 85 percent of 180 = 153
- 95 percent of 180 = 171

To sum up, the low end of her training range is 117–135; moderate range is 135–153; and high end, 153–171. This formula is safe for everyone, including older adults and those new to exercise.

The Karvonen method

The Karvonen or Heart Rate Reserve (HRR) method, factors in the resting heart rate (RHR) (*see p18*) and is appropriate for younger and fitter individuals. Suppose our 40-year-old with an estimated maximum heart rate

---

Rating exercise intensity by perceived exertion

A simple way to assess whether you are exercising hard enough to improve your cardio fitness is known as rating of perceived exertion (RPE). This involves rating exercise intensity on a scale of 1–10 according to your overall sense of exertion, combining all sensations and feelings of physical stress, effort, and fatigue.

Alternatively, or in addition, you can use the "talk test," which is a simple measure of intensity based on breathlessness alone. You should be able to talk, but not sing. If you can't talk, the intensity is too hard; if you can sing, it's too easy.

The following rating scale combines RPE with the talk test and with heart rate (HR) training ranges.

RPE 1   Very light; can sing out loud; non-exercise HR

RPE 2–3   Light; can talk easily; warm-up/recovery HR

RPE 4–5   Moderately easy; talking requires little effort; 40–50 percent HR

RPE 6–7   Somewhat hard to hard; talking requires some effort; 60–70 percent HR

RPE 8–9   Very hard; talking requires a lot of effort; 80–90 percent HR

RPE 10   Peak effort; no talking; 100 percent HR

---

of 180 has a resting heart rate of 70. The HRR is the difference between her EMHR and RHR: 180 minus 70 = 110. The formula is slightly complicated because first we take a percentage of her HRR and then add her RHR back in to arrive at her training range levels of 60–80 percent HRR. (Don't worry about the math—the chart opposite does the work for you.) Notice that the percentage levels are lower than in the previous example, because this formula yields a more aggressive training range.

Once you figure out your training range, a heart rate monitor is a valuable tool to use during exercise to make sure that you are working at the proper level.

Gearing up for fitness walking

All you really need is a good pair of walking shoes. Choose a pair with a firm heel cup for stability, supportive cushioning in the heel, flexible soles to enhance a smooth heel-to-toe motion, and plenty of room to spread out your toes in the push-off phase (you should be able to wiggle your toes freely).

Running shoes are not the best choice for walking because the cushioning is designed differently for pounding and high impact. The thick sole of the running shoe is too stiff for walking, may cause blisters, and can catch on small bumps in the road.

Be sure to try on walking shoes at the end of the day, when your feet may be slightly swollen, and wear the same weight socks you intend to use for walking. The shoes should feel good right out of the box: don't let a salesperson tell you to "break them in."

When it's very cold outside, cover your head and hands. Wear several light layers of clothing that you can easily add or remove en route. You should feel a slight chill when you first step outside; this will turn to a warm glow as you start to move. When you walk in the heat, stay cool by wearing light, loose clothing. Protect your skin from the sun and avoid the midday heat.

Remember to drink plenty of cool water before, during, and after your session—by the time you feel thirsty during a workout you are headed toward

Correct posture while walking

This minimizes the risk of injury and fatigue and maximizes benefits. Use core strength to keep the torso upright.

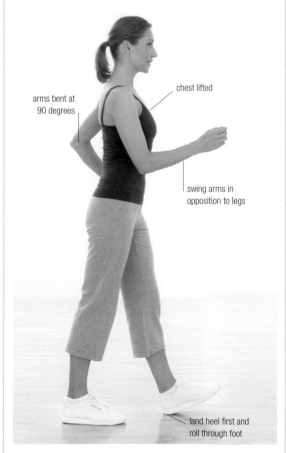

arms bent at 90 degrees

chest lifted

swing arms in opposition to legs

land heel first and roll through foot

Stand tall, with your head centered, your chin level, and your eyes forward. Lift your chest and relax your shoulders down and back. Contract your abdominals and maintain neutral spine alignment in the lower back. Bend your arms to 90 degrees.

Lower leg strengtheners for walking

The muscles in the lower legs need to be strengthened to keep up with the powerful muscles of the upper legs.

Heel-walking

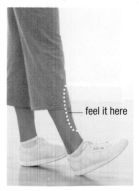

feel it here

Walking on your heels strengthens the tibialis anterior in the front of the shin and is a good drill for the heel strike.

Toe-walking

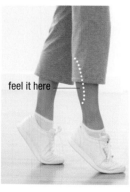

feel it here

Toe walking strengthens the gastrocnemius and soleus muscles in the calf and is a good drill for the push-off.

dehydration, which can affect both your performance and your health. Carry a water bottle and take four gulps every 20 minutes during long walks. When walking, muscle cramps and side stitches can cause discomfort. For cramps, stretch the muscle by increasing tension in the opposing muscle. For example, if you have a spasm in your calf, contract the muscles on the front of your lower leg by wedging your foot under something stationary or holding it down with your other heel, and try to flex the foot. In the case of a stitch, slow down, breathe deeply, and massage the area near your diaphragm.

Improving walking technique

The walking foot action involves a heel strike followed by rolling onto the ball of the foot and finishing with a strong push off the toes. Land naturally on your foot, heel first, then roll through heel to arch to ball of foot to toes—and push off to start another step.

Stride length will vary according to your physical build and your walking speed. To get some idea of your stride length, stand with feet together and lean forward from the ankles. As you begin to lose balance, swing one leg forward and notice where the foot strikes the ground. As you become more experienced and want to pick up the pace, you will have to shorten your stride length in order to increase your speed.

Develop your walking technique by practicing heel- and toe-walking (*see box opposite*). Alternate between the two, doing 10–20 steps of each. Finally, practice rolling through the whole foot, from heel to toe.

To increase your speed, work on the push-off phase of the foot action. Each time you step down, contact the ground with the heel, roll onto the ball of the foot, and vigorously push off the toes. It is common to pick up the foot too soon, thereby losing much of the acceleration advantage. Keep the foot in contact with the ground as long as possible. Add the arms, swinging them in opposition to the legs. To increase the walking pace, increase the speed of the arm swing. The legs will follow the cadence of the arms.

Post-walk stretching

Your workout is not over until after you've stretched and had a drink of water. Hold each stretch for 20–30 seconds without bouncing, repeating on both legs.

Quad stretch

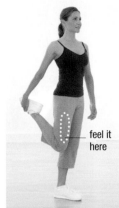

Stand on the left leg with the knee soft. Bend the right leg and, holding the foot or ankle, bring the heel toward the buttocks.

Hamstring stretch

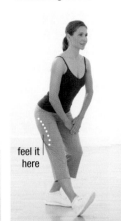

Stand on your left leg with the knee bent. Extend your right leg forward and rest the heel on the floor. Bend forward from the hip.

Calf stretch

feel it here

Take a giant step back with your right leg and press the heel into the floor. Bend your left leg, with the knee directly over the ankle.

Shin stretch

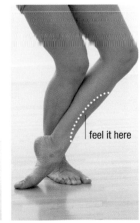

feel it here

Cross your left leg in front of your right with the top of your left foot on the floor. Bend your right leg to press into the left calf.

WALKING PROGRAM: 56–65

This program is designed for anyone who is new to exercise or who is returning to exercise after a long absence. The goal is to condition your cardiovascular system and muscles to physically adapt to the demands of the exercise. You will steadily build up to longer sessions at low-to-moderate intensity. Don't worry about how far or how fast you walk.

Health benefits of walking

Recent studies have shown that walking can reduce your risk of breast cancer, decrease intra-abdominal fat (associated with heart disease), lower the risk of hip fracture, and reduce back pain. Walking 30 minutes a day (combined with reducing television viewing to fewer than 10 hours a week) can significantly reduce new cases of obesity and diabetes. All of these health-related conditions can affect your body age by limiting your ability to function and maintain an active lifestyle.

Health experts recommend that every adult engage in a minimum of 30 minutes of moderate-intensity physical activity most days of the week. However, research shows that three 10-minute or two 15-minute periods provide about the same benefit, so you can accumulate your exercise in doses. If this works best for you, try to be consistent about the timing and establish a pattern: 10 minutes in the morning, 10 at lunchtime, and 10 in the evening. If you are already accumulating exercise during the day, you can build on what you are currently doing.

Fitting exercise into your life

To ensure a successful walking program, choose the best time of day for you and schedule it in. If you have time to walk in the morning, you are more likely to fit it in before the distractions of the day interfere. There will always be distractions, so do make exercise a priority.

Some people like to walk toward the end of the day to relieve tension and help digest their dinner. Light rhythmic exercise in the evening has a "tranquilizing" effect and a short stroll can help you sleep, but more vigorous exercise may be over-stimulating and may interfere with your sleep.

Walking is highly adaptable, with many options of where to exercise. If you walk on city streets, wear well-cushioned shoes and watch out for obstacles like pot-holes and broken curbs. In city parks, look for open areas and walk at peak times when there are other people around. Outdoor tracks have cushioned surfaces that are easy on the knees, and their measured distances make it easy to monitor pace. Indoor treadmills offer the advantage of a uniform, cushioned surface, adjustable for speed and incline, instant read-outs of time, distance, and calories, and protection from inclement weather.

Beginning to walk

• If you are a beginner, set a pace for your program and don't push yourself too hard to begin with.

• During Weeks 1–3, aim for an RPE of 2–3, which is a warm-up and recovery pace (see p145). In Week 4, when you increase the pace slightly to an RPE rating of 4–5, spend the first and last five minutes of your workout walking at the slower pace for your warm-up and cool-down.

• Reduce your pace if you find that you are unable to speak in a conversational tone, if it takes more than five minutes for your heart rate to slow down, or if you feel faint or have difficulty breathing.

• Be sure to do the basic walking stretches after every session (see p147).

56-65 8-week base-building program

Week	Monday	Tuesday	Wednesday	Thursday	Friday	Saturday	Sunday
1 15–18-minute workouts	15 mins RPE 2–3	15 mins RPE 2–3	15 mins RPE 2–3	18 mins RPE 2–3	18 mins RPE 2–3	18 mins RPE 2–3	Rest
2 20–22-minute workouts	20 mins RPE 2–3	20 mins RPE 2–3	20 mins RPE 2–3	22 mins RPE 2–3	22 mins RPE 2–3	22 mins RPE 2–3	Rest
3 25–30-minute workouts	25 mins RPE 2–3	25 mins RPE 2–3	25 mins RPE 2–3	30 mins RPE 2–3	30 mins RPE 2–3	30 mins RPE 2–3	Rest
4 15–18-minute workouts	15 mins RPE 4–5	15 mins RPE 4–5	15 mins RPE 4–5	18 mins RPE 4–5	18 mins RPE 4–5	18 mins RPE 4–5	Rest
5 20–22-minute workouts	20 mins RPE 4–5	20 mins RPE 4–5	20 mins RPE 4–5	22 mins RPE 4–5	22 mins RPE 4–5	22 mins RPE 4–5	Rest
6 25–28-minute workouts	25 mins RPE 4–5	25 mins RPE 4–5	25 mins RPE 4–5	28 mins RPE 4–5	28 mins RPE 4–5	28 mins RPE 4–5	Rest
7 -minute workouts	30 mins RPE 4–5	30 mins RPE 4–5	30 mins RPE 4–5	30 mins RPE 4–5	30 mins RPE 4–5	30 mins RPE 4–5	Rest
8 -minute workouts	40 mins RPE 4–5	40 mins RPE 4–5	40 mins RPE 4–5	40 mins RPE 4–5	40 mins RPE 4–5	40 mins RPE 4–5	Rest

RPE = rating of perceived exertion (*see p145*)

WALKING PROGRAM: 46–55

Once you have established a regular walking base and are walking for 30 minutes at RPE 4–5 six days a week (as in the 56–65 Walking Program on pp148–49), you are ready to pick up the pace. This program requires a measured distance, such as a high-school track, or any other set distance that you can use to compare your finish-time.

Benefits of aerobic exercise

Aerobic exercise is essential for weight loss and you will burn more calories by walking farther and faster. For example, a woman weighing 145lb (65.8kg) who walks for 30 minutes at a brisk pace of 4 miles per hour (mph) (6 kilometres per hour/kph) would burn about 157 calories; walking at a moderate pace of 3mph
(5kph), she would burn about 114 calories.

Sustained aerobic activities demand the greatest caloric expenditure. The rhythmic movement of the large muscle groups requires the body to expend a lot of calories to sustain the activity. One pound (45g) of body fat contains 3,500 calories. By increasing your exercise to burn 300 extra calories a day and by decreasing your daily diet by 200 calories or more, you can lose one pound (45g) of body fat per week.

Dieting alone works against healthy weight loss because it can lower the metabolism, increase the appetite, and reduce lean body mass. Conversely, exercise increases the metabolism, suppresses the appetite, and conserves muscle tissue. Weight loss from exercise is primarily fat loss; as you exercise regularly, you will reduce fat stores from the whole body, developing leaner, toned muscles instead. The gain in lean muscle tissue and loss of excess fat results in trimmer contours and smaller circumferences, regardless of the weight lost.

New research highlights another important health benefit of aerobic exercise: as you reduce your waistline, you are also fighting the deep visceral fat that surrounds your organs and increases your risk

of heart disease (see pp14–15). Not only will your clothing fit better and your self-image improve, but you will live longer to enjoy your new figure.

Warm-ups and cool-downs

Begin your workout by warming up for about five minutes. The best warm-up is to perform your activity (here, walking) slowly to prepare the muscles involved for more vigorous work. If you have time to stretch after your warm-up and before the main aerobic component, this is ideal. Otherwise, go right into your workout. Be sure to cool down for five minutes at the end by slowing your pace. After you finish, do your stretches (see pp150–51). If you have time to stretch only once, do it after completion of your workout.

Tips on moderate-to-brisk walking

• Bend your arms to 90 degrees and keep the elbows close to your body. Relax your hands in loose fists. Move the arms from the shoulders, not the elbows.

• Use a more forceful arm swing to increase tempo (to increase pace, simply increase the speed of the arm swing and the leg action will follow).

• Swing the arms forward and back like a pendulum (not side-to-side). Make sure your arms don't cross your body.

• To accelerate, shorten your stride. Take smaller, quicker steps and pump your arms.

• Focus on inhaling and exhaling rhythmically as you walk, synchronizing your breathing with your steps.

46-55 8-week moderate-to-brisk walking program

Week	Monday	Tuesday	Wednesday	Thursday	Friday	Saturday	Sunday
1 minute orkouts	Warm-up: 5 mins 1 mile (1.6km): 20 min Cool-down: 5 mins	Warm-up: 5 mins 1 mile (1.6km): 20 min Cool-down: 5 mins	Warm-up: 5 mins 1 mile (1.6km): 20 min Cool-down: 5 mins	Warm-up: 5 mins 1 mile (1.6km): 20 min Cool-down: 5 mins	Warm-up: 5 mins 1 mile (1.6km): 20 min Cool-down: 5 mins	Warm-up: 5 mins 1 mile (1.6km): 20 min Cool-down: 5 mins	Rest
2 minute orkouts	Warm-up: 5 mins 1.5 miles (2.4km): 30 mins Cool-down: 5 mins	Warm-up: 5 mins 1.5 miles (2.4km): 30 mins Cool-down: 5 mins	Warm-up: 5 mins 1.5 miles (2.4km): 30 mins Cool-down: 5 mins	Warm-up: 5 mins 1.5 miles (2.4km): 30 mins Cool-down: 5 mins	Warm-up: 5 mins 1.5 miles (2.4km): 30 mins Cool-down: 5 mins	Warm-up: 5 mins 1.5 miles (2.4km): 30 mins Cool-down: 5 mins	Rest
3 minute orkouts	Warm-up: 5 mins 2 miles (3.2km): 40 mins Cool-down: 5 mins	Warm-up: 5 mins 2 miles (3.2km): 40 mins Cool-down: 5 mins	Warm-up: 5 mins 2 miles (3.2km): 40 mins Cool-down: 5 mins	Warm-up: 5 mins 2 miles (3.2km): 40 mins Cool-down: 5 mins	Warm-up: 5 mins 2 miles (3.2km): 40 mins Cool-down: 5 mins	Warm-up: 5 mins 2 miles (3.2km): 40 mins Cool-down: 5 mins	Rest
4 minute orkouts	Warm-up: 5 mins 2 miles (3.2km): 38 mins Cool-down: 5 mins	Warm-up: 5 mins 2 miles (3.2km): 38 mins Cool-down: 5 mins	Warm-up: 5 mins 2 miles (3.2km): 38 mins Cool-down: 5 mins	Warm-up: 5 mins 2 miles (3.2km): 38 mins Cool-down: 5 mins	Warm-up: 5 mins 2 miles (3.2km): 38 mins Cool-down: 5 mins	Warm-up: 5 mins 2 miles (3.2km): 38 mins Cool-down: 5 mins	Rest
5 minute orkouts	Warm-up: 5 mins 2 miles (3.2km): 36 mins Cool-down: 5 mins	Warm-up: 5 mins 2 miles (3.2km): 36 mins Cool-down: 5 mins	Warm-up: 5 mins 2 miles (3.2km): 36 mins Cool-down: 5 mins	Warm-up: 5 mins 2 miles (3.2km): 36 mins Cool-down: 5 mins	Warm-up: 5 mins 2 miles (3.2km): 36 mins Cool-down: 5 mins	Warm-up: 5 mins 2 miles (3.2km): 36 mins Cool-down: 5 mins	Rest
6 minute orkouts	Warm-up: 5 mins 2 miles (3.2km): 34 mins Cool-down: 5 mins	Warm-up: 5 mins 2 miles (3.2km): 34 mins Cool-down: 5 mins	Warm-up: 5 mins 2 miles (3.2km): 34 mins Cool-down: 5 mins	Warm-up: 5 mins 2 miles (3.2km): 34 mins Cool-down: 5 mins	Warm-up: 5 mins 2 miles (3.2km): 34 mins Cool-down: 5 mins	Warm-up: 5 mins 2 miles (3.2km): 34 mins Cool-down: 5 mins	Rest
7 minute orkouts	Warm-up: 5 mins 2 miles (3.2km): 32 mins Cool-down: 5 mins	Warm-up: 5 mins 2 miles (3.2km): 32 mins Cool-down: 5 mins	Warm-up: 5 mins 2 miles (3.2km): 32 mins Cool-down: 5 mins	Warm-up: 5 mins 2 miles (3.2km): 32 mins Cool-down: 5 mins	Warm-up: 5 mins 2 miles (3.2km): 32 mins Cool-down: 5 mins	Warm-up: 5 mins 2 miles (3.2km): 32 mins Cool-down: 5 mins	Rest
8 minute orkouts	Warm-up: 5 mins 2 miles (3.2km): 30 mins Cool-down: 5 mins	Warm-up: 5 mins 2 miles (3.2km): 30 mins Cool-down: 5 mins	Warm-up: 5 mins 2 miles (3.2km): 30 mins Cool-down: 5 mins	Warm-up: 5 mins 2 miles (3.2km): 30 mins Cool-down: 5 mins	Warm-up: 5 mins 2 miles (3.2km): 30 mins Cool-down: 5 mins	Warm-up: 5 mins 2 miles (3.2km): 30 mins Cool-down: 5 mins	Rest

(km = kilometre)

WALKING PROGRAM: 36–45

To train your heart to work in the upper reaches of your training range (*see pp144–45*), you need to intensify the exercise. However, before attempting this program, which adds short, intense intervals into a more moderate pace of activity, you must have established a solid base of aerobic conditioning—such as the 46–55 program on pages 150–51.

Working in your training range

Optimal cardiovascular conditioning benefits occur when your heart is working in your training range. If your heart rate is too low, you are not working hard enough to produce a training effect; if your heart rate is too high, you will not be able to sustain the activity and will soon fatigue. As your fitness level improves, your body becomes more efficient and you can perform more work at a relatively lower heart rate.

Adding high-intensity intervals

Your intervals are determined by two factors: intensity and duration. You can increase the intensity by either picking up the pace or by walking up hills and inclines, which provides resistance.

You can use either a percentage of your heart rate training range or a corresponding RPE (*see p145*) as the measure of intensity.

A good rule-of-thumb for determining the pattern of the intervals is to rest for twice the length of the exertion. In other words, if you are doing one minute of high-intensity work, rest for two; two minutes at high intensity, rest for four, and so on.

Caution: most experts advise against using hand-held or ankle weights to increase the intensity while you walk because of the risk of straining the joints.

Benefits of high-intensity work

Working at the high end of your training range has additional health benefits. A recent study established a link between high-intensity exercise and longevity. If you are trying to lose weight, it is also a more

How the 36–45 walking program works
• Over the course of this program, which includes interval training, the duration of the workout increases. Week 1 starts with a 30-minute walk at a steady pace, RPE 6–7, and increases to a 50-minute workout in Week 8.
• The intensity of the workout also increases. On alternate days, we add interval training (IT), which consists of short segments of high-intensity and lower intensity work. For example, 1 minute at RPE 8–9, alternating with 2 minutes at RPE 4–5 in Week 1, increasing to 3 minutes at RPE 8–9, alternating with 6 minutes at RPE 4–5 in Week 4.
• Each IT session in this program starts with a 10-minute warm-up, consisting of 5 minutes at RPE 2–3, and 5 minutes at RPE 4–5. It ends with a 5-minute cool-down at RPE 2–3.

efficient way to burn calories—the more intense the activity, the more calories you burn per minute.

Power-walking technique

Use the following techniques when making the transition from moderate (3mph/5kph) or brisk (4mph/6kph) walking to power-walking (4.5–5mph/7–8kph):

• Take shorter, quicker steps.
• Focus on the push-off.
• Use quick, powerful arm swings.
• Lean forward slightly from the ankles (not the hips).
• Walk on an imaginary center line, as if you were on a tightrope.

36-45 8-week program of interval training & high intensity work

Week	Monday	Tuesday	Wednesday	Thursday	Friday	Saturday	Sunday
1 minute rkouts	30 mins steady pace, RPE 6–7	Warm-up: 10 mins + 5 intervals of 1 min, RPE 8–9, alternating with 2 mins, RPE 4–5 Cool-down: 5 mins	30 mins steady pace, RPE 6–7	Warm-up: 10 mins + 5 intervals of 1 min, RPE 8–9, alternating with 2 mins, RPE 4–5 Cool-down: 5 mins	30 mins steady pace, RPE 6–7	Warm-up: 10 mins + 5 intervals of 1 min, RPE 8–9, alternating with 2 mins, RPE 4–5 Cool-down: 5 mins	Rest
2 minute rkouts	30 mins steady pace, RPE 6–7	Warm-up: 10 mins + 5 intervals of 1 min, RPE 8–9, alternating with 2 mins, RPE 4–5 Cool-down: 5 mins	30 mins steady pace at RPE 6–7	Warm-up: 10 mins + 5 intervals of 1 min, RPE 8–9, alternating with 2 mins, RPE 4–5 Cool-down: 5 mins	30 mins steady pace, RPE 6–7	Warm-up: 10 mins + 5 intervals of 1 min, RPE 8–9, alternating with 2 mins, RPE 4–5 Cool-down: 5 mins	Rest
3 minute rkouts	45 mins steady pace, RPE 6–7	Warm-up: 10 mins + 5 intervals of 2 mins, RPE 8–9, alternating with 4 mins, RPE 4–5 Cool-down: 5 mins	45 mins steady pace, RPE 6–7	Warm-up: 10 mins + 5 intervals of 2 min, RPE 8–9, alternating with 4 mins, RPE 4–5 Cool-down: 5 mins	45 mins steady pace, RPE 6–7	Warm-up: 10 mins + 5 intervals of 2 mins, RPE 8–9, alternating with 4 mins, RPE 4–5 Cool-down: 5 mins	Rest
4 minute rkouts	45 mins steady pace, RPE 6–7	Warm-up: 10 mins + 5 intervals of 2 mins, RPE 8–9, alternating with 4 mins, RPE 4–5 Cool-down: 5 mins	45 mins steady pace, RPE 6–7	Warm-up: 10 mins + 5 intervals of 2 mins, RPE 8–9, alternating with 4 mins, RPE 4–5 Cool-down: 5 mins	45 mins steady pace, RPE 6–7	Warm-up: 10 mins + 5 intervals of 2 mins, RPE 8–9, alternating with 4 mins, RPE 4–5 Cool-down: 5 mins	Rest
5 minute rkouts	45 mins steady pace, RPE 6–7	Warm-up: 10 mins + 3 intervals of 3 mins, RPE 8–9, alternating with 6 mins, RPE 4–5 Cool-down: 5 mins	45 mins steady pace, RPE 6–7	Warm-up: 10 mins + 3 intervals of 3 mins, RPE 8–9, alternating with 6 mins, RPE 4–5 Cool-down: 5 mins	45 mins steady pace, RPE 6–7	Warm-up: 10 mins + 3 intervals of 3 mins, RPE 8–9, alternating with 6 mins, RPE 4–5 Cool-down: 5 mins	Rest
6 minute rkouts	45 mins steady pace, RPE 6–7	Warm-up: 10 mins + 3 intervals of 3 mins, RPE 8–9, alternating with 6 mins, RPE 4–5 Cool-down: 5 mins	45 mins steady pace, RPE 6–7	Warm-up: 10 mins + 3 intervals of 3 mins RPE 8–9, alternating with 6 mins, RPE 4–5 Cool-down: 5 mins	45 mins steady pace, RPE 6–7	Warm-up: 10 mins + 3 intervals of 3 mins, RPE 8–9, alternating with 6 mins, RPE 4–5 Cool-down: 5 mins	Rest
7 minute rkouts	50 mins steady pace, RPE 6–7	Warm-up: 10 mins + 4 intervals of 3 mins, RPE 8–9, alternating with 6 mins, RPE 4–5 Cool-down: 5 mins	50 mins steady pace, RPE 6–7	Warm-up: 10 mins + 4 intervals of 3 mins, RPE 8–9, alternsating with 6 mins, RPE 4–5 Cool-down: 5 mins	50 mins steady pace, RPE 6–7	Warm-up: 10 mins + 4 intervals of 3 mins, RPE 8–9, alternating with 6 mins, RPE 4–5 Cool-down: 5 mins	Rest
8 minute rkouts	50 mins steady pace, RPE 6–7	Warm-up: 10 mins + 4 intervals of 3 mins, RPE 8–9, alternating with 6 mins, RPE 4–5 Cool-down: 5 mins	50 mins steady pace, RPE 6–7	Warm-up: 10 mins + 4 intervals of 3 mins RPE 8–9, alternating with 6 mins, RPE 4–5 Cool-down: 5 mins	50 mins steady pace, RPE 6–7	Warm-up: 10 mins + 4 intervals of 3 mins, RPE 8–9, alternating with 6 mins, RPE 4–5 Cool-down: 5 mins	Rest

RPE = rating of perceived exertion (*see p145*)

WALKING PROGRAM: 26–35

If you have a well-established cardio routine, you will need to vary it if you want to continue to improve. No matter how fit you are, your body will eventually adapt to any kind of exercise, causing you to hit a plateau. Whether you are trying to shed some weight, get stronger, or advance your sports skills, the trick is to continuously challenge your body.

Changing your routine

When you do the same routine for more than a few months, the cardiovascular and muscular systems stop improving because they don't have to. At any level of fitness, however, you can boost your results by changing the FIT variables (see pp12–13) and/or the type of workout you are doing—for example, if you've been walking, try cycling or swimming instead. The technical name for this method is "periodization." Periodization applies to cycles of training (for instance, following one of the programs in this book for 8 weeks then moving to a different one) as well as to changing your daily routine, as in this walking program.

Boosting your results

Unlike cardio (aerobic) programs with a single focus, this program combines elements of distance, speed, and interval training. The mix of training factors provides the stimulus for change and can help you meet your goals, whether they are to reduce body fat, increase your cardiovascular endurance, or power up your walking speed.

Establishing your heart rate training ranges will be useful in determining the proper intensity for the different workouts. Figure out what your low, mid, and high ranges are, according to one of the two formulae described on page 144. Once you become familiar with taking your own pulse and associating it with your subjective feelings of exertion, you can quickly tune into the proper intensity. Just remember that as you become more conditioned, you will have to work harder to achieve the same level of exertion.

Following the 26–35 program

• As in the previous program (pp152–53), intervals of high- and low-intensity are incorporated into the workouts. In this program, however, the days on which IT sessions occur vary in order to prompt continued cardiovascular improvement.

• As in the previous program, each IT session starts with a 10-minute warm-up consisting of 5 minutes at RPE 2–3 and 5 minutes at RPE 4–5. Each IT session ends with a 5-minute cool-down at RPE 2–3.

• Once you you have reached a well-established fitness level, it is important to check that you are working at the correct level of intensity in order to continue improving cardiovascular fitness. A heart-rate monitor is a useful aid in ensuring that you continue challenging your cardiovascular system.

Exercise safely

Remember to allow ten minutes to warm up before you start and another five to cool down afterwards. It is best to cool down slowly after vigorous exercise— stopping abruptly may cause the blood to pool in your limbs, slowing its return to the brain and possibly causing dizziness or light-headedness. For a safe, comfortable recovery from strenuous exercise, continue light physical activity until your heart rate returns to below 120 beats per minute before you stop completely.

Caution: If you feel breathless, light-headed, or queasy after the workout, or if you experience undue fatigue or hunger, reduce the intensity of the exercise.

26–35 8-week program extending your cardio challenge

Week	Monday	Tuesday	Wednesday	Thursday	Friday	Saturday	Sunday
1 30–60-minute workouts	60 mins steady pace, RPE 6–7	Warm-up: 10 mins + 5 intervals of 1 min, RPE 8–9 alternating with 2 mins, RPE 4–5 Cool-down: 5 mins	45 mins steady pace, RPE 6–7	Warm-up: 10 mins + 5 intervals of 2 mins, RPE 8–9 alternating with 4 mins, RPE 4–5 Cool-down: 5 mins	60 mins steady pace, RPE 6–7	Warm-up: 10 mins + 5 intervals of 1 min, RPE 8–9 alternating with 2 mins, RPE 4–5 Cool-down: 5 mins	Rest
2 30–60-minute workouts	45 mins steady pace, RPE 6–7	60 mins steady pace, RPE 6–7	Warm-up: 10 mins + 5 intervals of 1 min, RPE 8–9 alternating with 2 mins, RPE 4–5 Cool-down: 5 mins	45 mins steady pace, RPE 6–7	Warm-up: 10 mins + 5 intervals of 2 mins, RPE 8–9 alternating with 4 mins, RPE 4–5 Cool-down: 5 mins	60 mins steady pace, RPE 6–7	Rest
3 30–60-minute workouts	Warm-up: 10 mins + 5 intervals of 1 min, RPE 8–9 alternating with 2 mins, RPE 4–5 Cool-down: 5 mins	45 mins steady pace, RPE 6–7	60 mins steady pace, RPE 6–7	Warm-up: 10 mins + 3 intervals of 3 mins, RPE 8–9 alternating with 6 mins, RPE 4–5 Cool-down: 5 mins	45 mins steady pace, RPE 6–7	Warm-up: 10 mins + 4 intervals of 3 mins, RPE 8–9 alternating with 6 mins, RPE 4–5 Cool-down: 5 mins	Rest
4 30–60-minute workouts	60 mins steady pace, RPE 6–7	45 mins steady pace, RPE 6–7	Warm-up: 10 mins + 5 intervals of 1 min, RPE 8–9 alternating with 2 mins, RPE 4–5 Cool-down: 5 mins	60 mins steady pace, RPE 6–7	Warm-up: 10 mins + 3 intervals of 3 mins, RPE 8–9 alternating with 6 mins, RPE 4–5 Cool-down: 5 mins	45 mins steady pace, RPE 6–7	Rest
5 30–60-minute workouts	Warm-up: 10 mins + 4 intervals of 3 mins, RPE 8–9 alternating with 6 mins, RPE 4–5 Cool-down: 5 mins	60 mins steady pace, RPE 6–7	45 mins steady pace, RPE 6–7	Warm-up: 10 mins + 5 intervals of 1 min, RPE 8–9 alternating with 2 mins, RPE 4–5 Cool-down: 5 mins	45 mins steady pace, RPE 6–7	60 mins steady pace, RPE 6–7	Rest
6 30–60-minute workouts	45 mins steady pace, RPE 6–7	Warm-up: 10 mins + 3 intervals of 3 mins, RPE 8–9 alternating with 6 mins, RPE 4–5 Cool-down: 5 mins	60 mins steady pace, RPE 6–7	Warm-up: 10 mins + 4 intervals of 3 mins, RPE 8–9 alternating with 6 mins, RPE 4–5 Cool-down: 5 mins	45 mins steady pace, RPE 6–7	Warm-up: 10 mins + 5 intervals of 1 min, RPE 8–9 alternating with 2 mins, RPE 4–5 Cool-down: 5 mins	Rest
7 30–60-minute workouts	60 mins steady pace, RPE 6–7	Warm-up: 10 mins + 5 intervals of 1 min, RPE 8–9 alternating with 2 mins, RPE 4–5 Cool-down: 5 mins	Warm-up: 10 mins + 4 intervals of 3 mins, RPE 8–9 alternating with 6 mins, RPE 4–5 Cool-down: 5 mins	45 mins steady pace, RPE 6–7	60 mins steady pace, RPE 6–7	Warm-up: 10 mins + 5 intervals of 2 mins, RPE 8–9 alternating with 4 mins, RPE 4–5 Cool-down: 5 mins	Rest
8 30–60-minute workouts	Warm-up: 10 mins + 3 intervals of 3 mins, RPE 8–9 alternating with 6 mins, RPE 4–5 Cool-down: 5 mins	60 mins steady pace, RPE 6–7	Warm-up: 10 mins + 5 intervals of 2 mins, RPE 8–9 alternating with 4 mins, RPE 4–5 Cool-down: 5 mins	60 mins steady pace, RPE 6–7	45 mins steady pace, RPE 6–7	Warm-up: 10 mins + 5 intervals of 1 min, RPE 8–9 alternating with 2 mins, RPE 4–5 Cool-down: 5 mins	Rest

RPE = rating of perceived exertion (*see p145*)

RESOURCES

For the US and Canada

Joan Pagano Fitness Group
401 East 89th Street (no. 2M)
New York, NY 10128, USA
Email: info@joanpaganofitness.
com
www.joanpaganofitness.com

YMCA of the USA
101 N. Wacker Drive
Chicago, IL 60606
www.ymca.net/
*Over 2,500 community-based
branches, providing health and
fitness programs for all ages.*

Fitness Wholesale
Tel (US): 1-888-FW-ORDER
Tel: 001-330-929-7227
email: fw@fwonline.com
www.fitnesswholesale.com
*For weights, a range of fitness
balls, including stability balls, tubes,
mats, and stretch bands.*

The Canadian Society for
Exercise Physiology
www.csep.ca/forms.asp
*Scientific authority on exercise
physiology, health, and fitness.*

For the UK

Totally Fitness
Tel: 020-7467-5929
email: sales@totallyfitness.com
www.totallyfitness.co.uk
*For weights, stability balls, stretch
bands, and resistance tubes.*

Newitt & Co Ltd
Tel: 01904-468551
email: sales@newitts.com
www.newitts.com
*For medicine balls, free weights,
ankle weights, and stretch bands.*

Sissel UK Limited
10 Moderna Business Park
Mytholmroyd, Halifax
West Yorkshire HX7 5RH
Tel: 01422 885433
email: info@sisseluk.com
www.sisseluk.com
*For gym mats, stability
balls (the Sissel Fitbox), and
stretch bands.*

New Balance Athletic Shoes
(UK) Ltd
320 Firecrest Court,
Centre Park, Warrington,
Cheshire WA1 1RG
Tel: 01925 423000
www.newbalance.co.uk
*For good walk-specific shoes and
excellent measuring service.*

Polar UK
Leisure Systems International Ltd
Northfield Road,
Southam
Warwickshire CV47 ORD
Tel: 01926 811611
www.polar-uk.com
Email: polarsd@lsi.co.uk
*For heart-rate monitors and
associated products*

National Osteoporosis Society
(NOS)
Camerton, Bath BA2 OPJ
Tel: 0845 130 3076 (general
enquiries)
Helpline (medical): 0845-
450 0230
email: info@nos.org.uk
www.nos.org.uk

The Ramblers' Association
2nd Floor, Camelford House
87–90 Albert Embankment
London SE1 7TW
Tel: 020 7339 8500
www.ramblers.org.uk
*Local groups, walking events,
and campaigns.*

For Australia

Elite Fitness Equipment
Tel: (In Australia only) 1800-622-
644
email: info@elitefitness.com.au
www.elitefitness.com.au

Fernwood Women's Health Club
National Office
Tel: (03) 5443-4555
Phone-a-club: 13-33-76
www.fernwoodfitness.com.au

Osteoporosis Australia
Level 1, 52 Parramatta Road
Forest Lodge
NSW 2037
Tel: (02) 9518-8140
www.osteoporosis.org.au

INDEX

ACKNOWLEDGMENTS

Author's acknowledgments

With special thanks to all who supported this effort—my family and friends, clients, and professional colleagues. To James for nurturing me with his love and cooking, my sister Lucy for jumping in when the going got rough, and my mother for giving me a sense of purpose. To Jackie for steering me in the right direction so many years ago. Thanks to my clients for their encouragement and guidance. And to my colleagues in both fitness and publishing for their enthusiasm and generosity of spirit.

Thanks to DK for putting together an amazing team. To Mary-Clare Jerram and Carl Raymond for the opportunity to produce this book and to Jenny Jones for her wise counsel. To Gillian Roberts behind the scenes. To Irene for her creative problem-solving and clever organizational skills, Miranda for her brilliant art direction, and Ruth for making the photos come to life. And to all of our gorgeous models who always said, "I'll try."

Publisher's acknowledgments

Dorling Kindersley would like to thank photographer Ruth Jenkinson and her assistants Sarah, Emma, Vicki, and Jono; Viv Riley at Touch Studios for helping to make everything go smoothly; models Resi Harris, Denny Kemp, Sheri Staplehurst, Sally Way; Roishin Donaghy for models' hair and makeup; Rebecca Markley for help at the photography sessions; Hilary Bird for the index; Sonia Charbonnier for all her DTP support. Special thanks to Totally Fitness (*see p156*) for lending us the stability ball. All images © DK Images. For more information see www.dkimages.com

Credits

The norms on pp25–26 were adapted from *YMCA Fitness Testing and Assessment Manual, 4th ed*. With permission of the YMCA of the USA, 101 N. Wacker Drive, Chicago, IL 60606.

ABOUT THE AUTHOR

Joan Pagano, a Phi Beta Kappa, cum laude graduate of Connecticut College, is certified in health and fitness instruction by the American College of Sports Medicine (ACSM), whose credentials provide the very best measure of competence as a professional. She has worked as a personal fitness trainer on Manhattan's Upper East Side since 1988, providing professional guidance and support to people at all levels of fitness. Through her work, she has created hundreds of training programs for individuals, groups, fitness facilities, schools, hospitals, and corporations.

Today, Joan manages her own staff of fitness specialists, who work together as Joan Pagano Fitness Group. For many years, she served as Director of the Personal Trainer Certification Program at Marymount Manhattan College, where she remains on the faculty as the instructor in fitness evaluation techniques. She is also a nationally recognized provider of continuing education courses for fitness trainers through IDEA (an organization that supports fitness professionals worldwide with education and career development).

Joan's knowledge of women's health issues evolved naturally from her work. Women trust Joan to guide them through periods of physical transition, such as pregnancy and childbirth or when fighting disease. As fitness consultant to SHARE, the breast cancer support group, she has worked with breast cancer survivors since 1992. Their concerns about menopause prompted Joan to study how exercise could help manage the side effects of this stage in life, and, in particular, how exercise could help fight osteoporosis. Now Joan is recognized by the industry as a leading authority on exercise program design strategies for osteoporosis.